THE ALPHA LIPOIC ACID BIBLE

An Essential Guide To Alpha Lipoic Acid: Benefits, Uses, And Its Powerful Effects On Aging And Wellbeing

DR. KYREN STEVEN

Table of Contents

CHAPTER ONE
Chemical Structure And Properties

Alpha Lipoic Acid (ALA), also known as thioctic acid, has a distinctive chemical structure and properties that contribute to its biological functions. Here's an overview:

Chemical Structure:

- **Structure**: Alpha Lipoic Acid is a dithiol compound, meaning it contains two sulfur atoms (in a disulfide bond) separated by a carbon atom.

- **Molecular Formula**: The molecular formula of ALA is $C_8H_{14}O_2S_2$.

- **Structure**: It consists of an octanoic acid molecule (an 8-carbon fatty acid) with a thiol group (-SH) attached at one end, and a carboxylic acid group (-COOH) at the other end.

Properties:

Introductory

Alpha Lipoic Arcid (ALA) is a naturally occurring compound that functions as a coenzyme in several important metabolic reactions in the body. Here are some key points about ALA:

- **Natural Compound**: ALA is synthesized in small amounts by the human body and can also be consumed through certain foods.

- **Antioxidant Properties**: One of its primary roles is as an antioxidant, which means it helps neutralize harmful free radicals in the body. This property is beneficial in combating oxidative stress and protecting cells from damage.

- **Metabolic Functions**: ALA plays a crucial role in energy production within cells. It is involved in the metabolism of carbohydrates, fats, and proteins, converting nutrients into energy that the body can use.

- **Regeneration of Antioxidants**: ALA is unique in its ability to regenerate other antioxidants such as vitamin C, vitamin E, and glutathione after they have neutralized free radicals. This makes it a valuable compound in maintaining a balanced antioxidant system in the body.

- **Potential Health Benefits**: Due to its antioxidant properties and role in cellular metabolism, ALA has been studied for its potential health benefits. It may support nerve health, cardiovascular health, and skin health. Some research also suggests it may help with blood sugar regulation and reducing inflammation.

- **Sources**: ALA is found naturally in small amounts in foods such as spinach, broccoli, yeast, liver, and kidney. It is also available as a dietary supplement.

- **Supplement Use**: ALA suppleme sometimes used to complement a heal especially in conditions where ant support or metabolic regulation is However, like any supplement, its use be discussed with a healthcare prov determine appropriateness and dosage.

Overall, Alpha Lipoic Acid is recogn its versatile roles in metabolisr antioxidant defense, contributing potential health benefits across systems in the body.

• **Water and Fat Solubility**: ALA is unique in that it is both water-soluble and fat-soluble (lipophilic). This allows it to function effectively in both aqueous and lipid environments within cells.

• **Antioxidant Activity**: ALA exhibits potent antioxidant properties due to its ability to neutralize free radicals. It can directly scavenge reactive oxygen species (ROS) and also regenerate other antioxidants such as vitamin C, vitamin E, and glutathione.

• **Metabolic Functions**: ALA plays a crucial role in energy metabolism. It is involved in mitochondrial function and the Krebs cycle (citric acid cycle), where it helps convert nutrients such as glucose into usable energy (ATP).

• **Chelation**: ALA can chelate (bind to) certain metal ions such as iron and copper, which can reduce their potentially harmful effects in the body.

• **Reduction Potential**: It has a relatively high reduction potential, which means it readily accepts and donates electrons, a property essential for its antioxidant function.

• **Stability**: ALA is stable under normal physiological conditions but can be metabolized in the liver and excreted in the urine after performing its antioxidant and metabolic functions.

Biological Functions:

• **Antioxidant Defense**: Protects cells from oxidative damage by neutralizing free radicals and regenerating other antioxidants.

• **Energy Production**: Facilitates the conversion of carbohydrates, fats, and proteins into energy.

- **Neuroprotection**: Shows potential in supporting nerve health and function.

- **Anti-inflammatory Effects**: May help reduce inflammation through its antioxidant actions.

Sources:

• ALA is naturally found in small amounts in foods such as spinach, broccoli, yeast, liver, and kidney. It is also available as a dietary supplement, often in the form of ALA or its more bioavailable form, R-alpha-lipoic acid (R-ALA).

Alpha Lipoic Acid's chemical structure and properties make it a versatile compound with antioxidant, metabolic, and potentially therapeutic benefits in various health conditions.

Antioxidant Properties & Role In Energy Metabolism

Alpha Lipoic Acid (ALA) possesses notable antioxidant properties and plays a crucial role in energy metabolism within the body. Let's delve into each of these aspects:

Antioxidant Properties:

• **Scavenging Free Radicals**: ALA acts as a potent antioxidant by neutralizing harmful free radicals. Free radicals are highly reactive molecules that can damage cells and contribute to aging and various diseases. ALA's ability to donate electrons allows it to neutralize these radicals, thereby protecting cells from oxidative stress.

• **Regeneration of Other Antioxidants**: One of ALA's unique features is its ability to regenerate other antioxidants such as vitamin C, vitamin E, and glutathione after they have neutralized free radicals. This recycling process helps maintain a robust antioxidant defense system in the body.

• **Protection Against Oxidative Stress**: By reducing oxidative stress, ALA may help mitigate cellular damage and inflammation associated with conditions like cardiovascular disease, diabetes, neurodegenerative disorders, and aging.

• **Metal Chelation**: ALA can chelate (bind to) metal ions such as iron and copper, which can reduce their pro-oxidant effects and further contribute to its antioxidant properties.

Role in Energy Metabolism:

• **Mitochondrial Function**: ALA plays a vital role in mitochondrial function, which is crucial for energy production in cells. Mitochondria are organelles responsible for generating ATP (adenosine triphosphate), the primary energy currency of the cell. ALA facilitates the transport of nutrients into mitochondria and enhances their conversion into ATP through the citric acid cycle (Krebs cycle).

• **Coenzyme Activity**: ALA functions as a coenzyme for several mitochondrial enzymes involved in energy metabolism. It helps activate enzymes like pyruvate dehydrogenase and alpha-ketoglutarate dehydrogenase, which are essential for converting carbohydrates and amino acids into energy.

• **Insulin Sensitivity**: ALA has been shown to improve insulin sensitivity in cells, which is important for glucose uptake and utilization. Enhanced insulin sensitivity can contribute to better energy metabolism and may benefit individuals with insulin resistance or type 2 diabetes.

• **Neuroprotective Effects**: The role of ALA in energy metabolism is also critical for maintaining proper function and health of the nervous system. It supports nerve cell function and may protect against oxidative damage in neurons, contributing to its potential neuroprotective effects.

Sources and Supplementation:

• ALA is naturally found in foods such as spinach, broccoli, yeast, liver, and kidney, albeit in small amounts. It is also available as a dietary supplement, often in the form of R-alpha-lipoic acid (R-ALA), which is more bioavailable than the synthetic S-alpha-lipoic acid.

Alpha Lipoic Acid's antioxidant properties and role in energy metabolism make it a valuable compound for overall health and well-being, potentially offering benefits in combating oxidative stress-related diseases and supporting cellular energy production.

Interaction with other antioxidants (e.g., vitamins C and E)

Alpha Lipoic Acid (ALA) interacts with other antioxidants like vitamins C and E in several beneficial ways due to its unique chemical properties and biological functions. Here's how ALA interacts with these antioxidants:

Regeneration of Other Antioxidants:

Vitamin C (Ascorbic Acid):

• ALA has the ability to regenerate oxidized vitamin C back to its active antioxidant form. After vitamin C neutralizes a free radical by donating an electron, it becomes oxidized. ALA can donate electrons to restore vitamin C to its antioxidant state, allowing it to continue its antioxidant role in the body.

• This recycling process helps prolong the antioxidant capacity of vitamin C and maintains its effectiveness in combating oxidative stress.

Vitamin E (Alpha-Tocopherol):

• Similar to vitamin C, ALA can regenerate vitamin E after it has neutralized a free radical. Vitamin E, being a fat-soluble antioxidant, protects cell membranes from lipid peroxidation caused by free radicals.

• ALA's ability to recycle vitamin E ensures that it remains active and available for continuous protection of cell membranes against oxidative damage.

Synergistic Antioxidant Effects:

• **Enhanced Antioxidant Defense**: ALA, vitamin C, and vitamin E together form a powerful antioxidant network. While ALA regenerates vitamins C and E, these vitamins in turn can also enhance ALA's own antioxidant activity. This synergy helps amplify the overall antioxidant defense system in the body, providing comprehensive protection against oxidative stress.

Practical Implications:

• **Combination Supplements**: Supplements that combine ALA with vitamins C and E are available and may offer enhanced antioxidant benefits. These combinations are often used in formulations aimed at supporting overall antioxidant status and combating oxidative damage associated with aging, inflammation, and various diseases.

• **Health Benefits**: The combined use of ALA with vitamins C and E may potentially improve cardiovascular health, support immune function, and protect against neurodegenerative diseases by reducing oxidative damage to cells and tissues.

Considerations:

- **Dosage and Balance**: While synergistic effects are beneficial, it's essential to consider the appropriate dosage and balance of these antioxidants. Excessive antioxidant supplementation may have unintended effects, and individual needs vary based on factors like age, health status, and diet.

- **Consultation with Healthcare Providers**: Before starting any new supplement regimen, especially one involving multiple antioxidants, it's advisable to consult with a healthcare provider. They can provide personalized recommendations based on individual health needs and potential interactions with medications.

Alpha Lipoic Acid's ability to regenerate vitamins C and E underscores its role in maintaining a robust antioxidant defense system.

This interaction highlights the importance of a balanced intake of antioxidants for overall health and protection against oxidative stress-related damage.

CHAPTER TWO
Health Benefits Of Alpha Lipoic Acid

Alpha Lipoic Acid (ALA) offers a variety of potential health benefits, primarily due to its antioxidant properties and roles in cellular metabolism. Here are some of the key health benefits associated with ALA:

• ALA is a potent antioxidant that scavenges free radicals and protects cells from oxidative stress. This oxidative stress, caused by an imbalance between free radicals and antioxidants in the body, is linked to various chronic diseases and aging processes. ALA's ability to neutralize free radicals and regenerate other antioxidants like vitamins C and E helps reduce oxidative damage to cells and tissues.

• ALA has been shown to enhance insulin sensitivity in cells, which can improve glucose uptake and utilization. This is particularly beneficial for individuals with insulin resistance or type 2 diabetes. By improving insulin sensitivity, ALA may help lower blood sugar levels and reduce the risk of complications associated with diabetes.

• ALA crosses the blood-brain barrier and has neuroprotective effects. It helps protect neurons from oxidative damage, which is implicated in neurodegenerative diseases such as Alzheimer's and Parkinson's disease. ALA's ability to regenerate antioxidants in the brain and its anti-inflammatory properties contribute to its potential neuroprotective benefits.

• **ALA may support cardiovascular health through several mechanisms:** It helps improve endothelial function, which is important for blood vessel health. ALA can reduce oxidative stress in the cardiovascular system, potentially lowering the risk of atherosclerosis and heart disease. It may also improve lipid profiles by reducing LDL cholesterol levels and increasing HDL cholesterol levels.

• Inflammation plays a key role in many chronic diseases, including cardiovascular disease, diabetes, and arthritis. ALA has anti-inflammatory properties that can help reduce inflammation markers and cytokine levels in the body. This anti-inflammatory action contributes to its overall health benefits.

• ALA has been studied for its potential benefits in promoting skin health and reducing signs of aging. As an antioxidant, ALA helps protect skin cells from oxidative damage caused by sun exposure and environmental pollutants. It may also support collagen production, which is essential for skin elasticity and hydration.

• Some studies suggest that ALA supplementation may aid in weight loss efforts by improving metabolic rate and increasing energy expenditure. It may also help regulate appetite and reduce oxidative stress associated with obesity.

• ALA has hepatoprotective properties, meaning it helps protect the liver from damage caused by toxins, alcohol, and certain medications. It supports liver function by reducing oxidative stress and inflammation in liver cells.

Dosage and Considerations:

• **Dosage**: Typical doses of ALA used in studies range from 300 mg to 600 mg per day, although higher doses may be used under medical supervision for specific conditions.

• **Safety**: ALA is generally considered safe when taken orally at recommended doses. However, like any supplement, it may interact with medications or have adverse effects in some individuals. Consultation with a healthcare provider is advisable before starting ALA supplementation, especially for those with existing medical conditions or taking medications.

Alpha Lipoic Acid offers a range of potential health benefits, particularly through its antioxidant properties, impact on insulin sensitivity, neuroprotection, cardiovascular support, and anti-inflammatory effects. Ongoing research continues to explore its therapeutic potential in various health conditions.

Clinical Applications In ALA In Diabetic Neuropathy Treatment

Alpha Lipoic Acid (ALA) has shown promise in the treatment of diabetic neuropathy, a common complication of diabetes characterized by nerve damage that can lead to symptoms such as pain, numbness, and tingling in the extremities. Here are the clinical applications of ALA in diabetic neuropathy treatment:

1. Antioxidant and Neuroprotective Effects:

• **Reduction of Oxidative Stress**: ALA's potent antioxidant properties help reduce oxidative stress in nerve cells. Diabetes is associated with increased oxidative stress, which contributes to nerve damage. ALA scavenges free radicals and regenerates other antioxidants, thereby protecting nerves from oxidative damage.

• **Neuroprotection**: ALA crosses the blood-brain barrier and accumulates in nerves, where it exerts neuroprotective effects. It enhances nerve blood flow and promotes the function and regeneration of nerve fibers.

2. Improved Nerve Function:

• **Symptomatic Relief**: ALA has been shown to improve symptoms of diabetic neuropathy such as pain, burning sensations, numbness, and tingling. Clinical trials have demonstrated that ALA supplementation can lead to a reduction in neuropathic symptoms and an improvement in nerve conduction velocity.

• **Quality of Life**: By alleviating neuropathic symptoms, ALA can significantly improve the quality of life for individuals with diabetic neuropathy, reducing pain and discomfort associated with the condition.

3. Regulation of Glucose Metabolism:

• **Enhanced Insulin Sensitivity**: ALA improves insulin sensitivity and glucose utilization in cells, which is beneficial for individuals with diabetes. Better glucose control can help mitigate nerve damage and reduce the progression of neuropathy.

4. Clinical Evidence and Recommendations:

• **Clinical Trials**: Several clinical studies have evaluated the efficacy of ALA in diabetic neuropathy treatment. Research, including meta-analyses, has shown that ALA supplementation at doses ranging from 600 mg to 1800 mg per day can improve neuropathic symptoms and nerve function.

• **Guidelines and Recommendations**: Based on evidence from clinical trials, some guidelines recommend ALA as a treatment option for diabetic neuropathy, particularly in cases where standard therapies are insufficient or intolerable.

5. Practical Considerations:

• **Duration of Treatment**: ALA treatment for diabetic neuropathy is often long-term to maintain symptom relief and neuroprotection.

Regular monitoring by healthcare providers is essential to assess the effectiveness and adjust the treatment regimen as needed.

• **Safety and Side Effects**: ALA is generally well-tolerated, but potential side effects such as gastrointestinal upset and skin rash may occur. High doses of ALA should be used cautiously, especially in individuals with existing medical conditions or taking other medications.

Alpha Lipoic Acid (ALA) has emerged as a valuable therapeutic option in the management of diabetic neuropathy due to its antioxidant properties, neuroprotective effects, and ability to improve nerve function and symptoms. While more research is needed to fully elucidate its mechanisms and long-term effects, ALA offers promise in enhancing the quality of life for individuals suffering from diabetic neuropathy.

Clinical Applications In Use In Metabolic Syndrome And Obesity

Alpha Lipoic Acid (ALA) has garnered interest for its potential applications in managing metabolic syndrome and obesity, two interconnected conditions that involve a cluster of metabolic abnormalities. Here's how ALA is being explored in clinical settings for these purposes:

1. Improving Insulin Sensitivity:

• **Mechanism**: ALA has been shown to improve insulin sensitivity in cells, which is crucial for regulating blood sugar levels. In individuals with metabolic syndrome or obesity, insulin resistance is a key feature where cells become less responsive to insulin, leading to elevated blood sugar levels.

• **Clinical Evidence**: Studies have demonstrated that ALA supplementation can enhance insulin action and glucose uptake in skeletal muscle and adipose tissue. This improvement in insulin sensitivity can help lower blood glucose levels and reduce the risk of type 2 diabetes.

2. Reducing Oxidative Stress:

• **Antioxidant Properties**: ALA acts as a potent antioxidant, scavenging free radicals and reducing oxidative stress. Oxidative stress is elevated in individuals with metabolic syndrome and obesity due to increased production of reactive oxygen species (ROS). ALA's antioxidant effects help protect cells from oxidative damage.

• **Clinical Evidence**: Research has shown that ALA supplementation can lower markers of oxidative stress and inflammation in patients with metabolic syndrome and obesity. This reduction in oxidative stress may contribute to improvements in metabolic parameters and overall health.

3. Weight Management:

• **Metabolic Effects**: ALA may influence metabolic processes that affect weight management. It has been suggested to enhance energy metabolism and increase energy expenditure, potentially aiding in weight loss efforts.

• **Clinical Evidence**: Some studies have explored the effects of ALA supplementation on body weight and fat mass in obese individuals. While results have been mixed, ALA's role in improving metabolic parameters such as lipid profiles and insulin sensitivity may indirectly support weight management efforts.

4. Cardiovascular Health:

• **Protective Effects**: ALA's antioxidant and anti-inflammatory properties may benefit cardiovascular health in individuals with metabolic syndrome or obesity. It can help improve endothelial function, reduce lipid oxidation, and lower blood pressure, all of which contribute to cardiovascular risk reduction.

• **Clinical Evidence**: Research suggests that ALA supplementation may improve vascular function and reduce markers of cardiovascular risk in obese and metabolic syndrome patients. These effects highlight ALA's potential as a supportive therapy for cardiovascular health in these populations.

5. Practical Considerations:

• **Dosage and Duration**: Typical doses of ALA used in clinical studies for metabolic syndrome and obesity range from 300 mg to 1800 mg per day. The duration of supplementation varies, but long-term use may be necessary to achieve and maintain beneficial effects.

- **Combination Therapies**: ALA is sometimes used in combination with other supplements or medications targeting metabolic syndrome components, such as diabetes medications or lipid-lowering agents. This combination approach may provide synergistic benefits in managing metabolic abnormalities.

Alpha Lipoic Acid (ALA) shows promise in clinical applications for managing metabolic syndrome and obesity by improving insulin sensitivity, reducing oxidative stress, supporting weight management, and potentially benefiting cardiovascular health. While more research is needed to fully establish its efficacy and safety, ALA represents a complementary approach to traditional therapies in addressing these complex metabolic conditions. As always, consulting with healthcare providers is recommended to determine the appropriate

use of ALA based on individual health needs
and conditions.

CHAPTER THREE
Potential Applications In Cancer Treatment

Alpha Lipoic Acid (ALA) has been studied for its potential applications in cancer treatment, although research in this area is still preliminary and ongoing. Here are some potential ways ALA may be applied in cancer treatment:

1. Antioxidant and Cytoprotective Effects:

• **Antioxidant Properties**: ALA is a potent antioxidant that helps neutralize free radicals and reduce oxidative stress. In the context of cancer, oxidative stress can contribute to cellular damage and promote tumor growth. ALA's antioxidant activity may help protect healthy cells from oxidative damage induced by cancer treatments such as chemotherapy and radiation therapy.

type, stage, treatment regimen, and overall health status.

Alpha Lipoic Acid (ALA) shows promise in cancer treatment primarily through its antioxidant, anti-inflammatory, and potentially sensitizing effects on cancer cells. While preliminary findings are encouraging, more rigorous clinical research is necessary to establish its efficacy, safety, and precise role in cancer therapy.

Neuroprotective Effects In Neurodegenerative Diseases

Alpha Lipoic Acid (ALA) has demonstrated significant potential as a neuroprotective agent in the context of neurodegenerative diseases. Here's how ALA exerts its neuroprotective effects and its implications in conditions like Alzheimer's disease, Parkinson's disease, and other neurodegenerative disorders:

Mechanisms of Neuroprotection:

Antioxidant Properties:

• ALA is a potent antioxidant that crosses the blood-brain barrier and accumulates in neural tissues. It scavenges free radicals and reduces oxidative stress, which is a key contributor to neuronal damage and death in neurodegenerative diseases.

Regeneration of Other Antioxidants:

• ALA can regenerate other antioxidants such as vitamin C, vitamin E, and glutathione after they have neutralized free radicals. This antioxidant recycling capability helps maintain a robust antioxidant defense system in the brain, protecting neurons from oxidative damage.

Anti-inflammatory Effects:

• Chronic inflammation is implicated in the progression of neurodegenerative diseases. ALA exhibits anti-inflammatory properties by modulating inflammatory pathways and reducing the production of pro-inflammatory molecules in the brain.

Metal Chelation:

• ALA can chelate (bind to) metal ions such as iron and copper, which can reduce their ability to catalyze oxidative reactions and generate free radicals in the brain. This metal-chelating activity contributes to ALA's neuroprotective effects.

Mitochondrial Support:

• ALA plays a role in mitochondrial function, enhancing energy production and maintaining mitochondrial health in neurons. Dysfunction of mitochondria is observed in many neurodegenerative diseases, and ALA's support of mitochondrial function can help preserve neuronal viability.

Neurodegenerative Diseases:

Alzheimer's Disease:

• ALA has been studied for its potential to mitigate Alzheimer's disease pathology. It may help reduce amyloid-beta accumulation, tau protein phosphorylation, and neuronal inflammation associated with Alzheimer's disease progression. Clinical studies have shown mixed results, but there is ongoing interest in ALA's role as an adjunct therapy.

Parkinson's Disease:

• Research suggests that ALA may protect dopaminergic neurons in the substantia nigra, which are affected in Parkinson's disease. ALA's antioxidant and anti-inflammatory properties may help mitigate oxidative stress and inflammation in Parkinson's disease models, potentially slowing disease progression.

Other Neurodegenerative Disorders:

• ALA has also been investigated in other neurodegenerative disorders such as Huntington's disease, amyotrophic lateral sclerosis (ALS), and multiple sclerosis (MS). While research is still in early stages, ALA's neuroprotective mechanisms make it a subject of interest for potential therapeutic applications in these conditions.

Clinical Applications and Considerations:

• **Supplementation**: ALA is available as a dietary supplement and is generally well-tolerated at recommended doses. Typical doses used in studies range from 600 mg to 1200 mg per day, although higher doses may be used under medical supervision for specific conditions.

• **Combination Therapies**: ALA is sometimes used in combination with other antioxidants or medications targeting neurodegenerative pathways. This approach aims to enhance therapeutic efficacy and address multiple aspects of disease pathology.

• **Consultation with Healthcare Providers**: As with any supplement, individuals considering ALA supplementation for neuroprotection should consult with healthcare providers, especially if they have underlying health conditions or are taking medications.

Alpha Lipoic Acid (ALA) holds promise as a neuroprotective agent in neurodegenerative diseases due to its antioxidant, anti-inflammatory, and mitochondrial-supporting properties. While more research is needed to establish its efficacy and optimal use in clinical settings, ALA represents a potential adjunct therapy for preserving neuronal function and mitigating neurodegenerative processes.

Common Side Effects & Interactions With Medications

Alpha Lipoic Acid (ALA) is generally considered safe when taken at appropriate doses, but like any supplement or medication, it can potentially cause side effects and interactions with certain medications. Here are the common side effects and interactions associated with ALA:

Common Side Effects:

•   **Gastrointestinal Upset**: Mild gastrointestinal symptoms such as nausea, vomiting, diarrhea, or stomach discomfort may occur, especially at higher doses.

• **Skin Rash**: Some individuals may experience allergic reactions or skin rash after taking ALA. This is more likely in those who are sensitive to sulfur-containing compounds.

• **Hypoglycemia**: ALA may lower blood sugar levels, particularly in individuals with diabetes or those taking medications to lower blood sugar. Monitoring blood glucose levels closely is important, especially when initiating ALA supplementation.

• **Insomnia**: Rarely, ALA may cause difficulty sleeping (insomnia) in some individuals.

in the regulation of glucose metabolism and the enhancement of insulin sensitivity.

• **Neurological Health:** ALA exhibits neuroprotective effects, which may be beneficial for conditions such as diabetic neuropathy and neurodegenerative diseases by supporting nerve function.

• **Safety and Considerations:** Although ALA is generally well-tolerated, it can interact with specific medications and may lower blood sugar levels, necessitating caution in individuals with diabetes or those taking related medications. Individuals with specific medical conditions, infants, pregnant or breastfeeding women, and special populations should consult with healthcare providers prior to use.

• **Integrating ALA into Your Diet and Supplements:** Although therapeutic doses are typically accomplished through supplementation, ALA can be incorporated into your diet through foods such as broccoli and spinach. It enhances the overall health benefits by complementing other antioxidants and supplements, such as vitamin C, vitamin E, and CoQ10.

• **Healthcare Provider Consultation:** It is imperative to consult with healthcare providers prior to initiating ALA supplementation, particularly if you are taking medications or have underlying health conditions. They are capable of offering customized recommendations that are tailored to your unique health requirements and objectives.

The potential of Alpha Lipoic Acid to support a variety of health and well-being aspects is promising. Individuals can make informed decisions to incorporate ALA into their health regimens in a safe and effective manner by comprehending its benefits, interactions, and optimal use.

THE END

www.ingramcontent.com/pod-product-compliance
Lightning Source LLC
Chambersburg PA
CBHW061306250726
48653CB00002B/797

Chapter One

A TINY FLARE in the back of her mind set Eunny Song's eye twitching. She flinched, nearly burning herself upon the heated end of the fire iron on her workbench. The thin sheet of wood she'd been attempting—badly—to burn with a decorative design ended up with a smoldering hole instead.

"Gods all break," Eunny muttered, tossing the ruined piece onto the bench. She'd never been much of a woodworker in any form, much less a hand at pyrography. Either she'd have to pass the repair job on to one of the regulars who came by Song's Scrap or see if the customer for the wood panels would accept a simpler job. The name of her shop should've said it all: scrap. Practical repairs that gave extra life to used objects and materials. Not art. She wasn't running a gallery. Wasn't running much of a repair café, either, if she were being honest with herself. Not a successful one, at any rate.

Eunny's eye twitched again. She bit her lip, fingers grazing the outer edge of the jittery skin. The small spasms had become a recurring theme over the last couple of weeks, or had it been a month already? Maybe even longer. They'd been so sporadic at first it was hard to remember the true start. The twitches coupled with a sense of restlessness that had been building in her chest. An intangible feeling of...certainty. Certainty without substance. All she knew was that whatever *it* was, it was coming, but it was still too nebulous for her to grasp.

She pushed back from her bench. Trudged past the stacks of items in need of repair, which had steadily been growing all summer, taking up more and more of her already limited space: tools that were more rust than metal, furniture missing arms or legs, fabric that even the moths and the rats found below their standards.

Junk. She would publicly deny it, but her repair café had descended to the depths of a glorified junk shop. Half of it wasn't even for pending jobs but "donations." The rest was work demanding more skill than she possessed to fulfill the owner's request. Demands for "pretty" rather than "functional".

"Shit." The curse hissed through her teeth as she tripped over a fallen handle of—something. Could've been a broom or a rake once. Hard to tell with its head missing. It was just a stick now, waiting to be repurposed, once the edges were re-sanded and polished so it wasn't just a length of splinters. It had fallen from the crate of Sylveren University's incomplete greenhouse order crammed into a corner as she dealt with it piecemeal.

Eunny started to jam the handle back into the crate, then took it back to the workbench instead. She could seal the crack near the end quick enough, give it a kiss with her sanding block and slap some wax on it. Done and done. Not up to her old standards, but the university was sending someone for pick-up later anyway, and they were already getting a partial order back. She could chuck it in with the few refurbished tool heads she'd managed to fix and the repaired seed trays, and that was one less thing cluttering up her place and her to-do list. Although, gods, if Gransen broke his temporary banishment and came to get the university's order—and saw how Eunny had made negligible progress on it... She could practically hear the café's self-professed "manager's" disapproval already.

Dodging the array of containers scavenged to collect drips from too many worn spots in the café's roof, Eunny made her way toward the back door. Rain in the somewhat notorious Valley of Sylveren was the normal order of things. Most days, Eunny loved it. The wind and the rain, the cloudy gray skies, the massive storm-colored lake and the verdant hills that surrounded the small town of Sylvan. It was home, far more than Graelynd, the neighboring country along the Valley's southern border, had ever been growing up. Even the towers and stone of Sylveren University set into the mountainside, its halls little more than a memory.

Everything fit. She belonged to the Valley. Had felt its claim when she was still just a child coming up for visits at her auntie's tea shop. Had felt the subtle shift in her head, her heart, of being welcomed beneath its oft-gray skies. The Valley of Sylveren didn't take to everyone. Most were merely tolerated, some outright rejected, plagued by a subtle—or not-so-subtle —feeling of unease. Of being repelled. But those the Valley found agreeable, it claimed. For so long, the knowledge that Eunny was amongst the latter had been a comfort.

Not so much these days. These last few... years.

Eunny shook her head, banishing the morose thoughts. The unseasonably deep, unrelenting gray was getting to her. She missed her best friend, Dae. Although Dae had only come to the Valley for a year of study at Sylveren University, Eunny had so quickly grown accustomed to having her friend in the flesh after years of long distance and letters. With Dae off doing her Adept Two research, fighting the poison devastating the northern kingdom of Rhell's landscape, their friendship had reverted to correspondence once again.

Eunny glanced up at the dark sky. Rain might be the norm here, but this was just excessive. It had been nearly two months since the summer solstice, and they hadn't seen consecutive days of dry moments, let alone blue sky. The Valley felt like a haven of mud more than anything else. Song's Scrap wasn't the only building in town struggling, but hers was a problem that required more than a recast of some waterproofing charms or quick patches to the shingles.

She paused on the outer stairwell that led to the loft above her aunt's beloved tearoom, the Mighty Leaf. Grimaced at the glaring, visible sags in her repair café's roof. Couldn't find any humor in the irony of a repair café in a state of disrepair itself. She turned away rather than keep looking at the temporary joins where the café had been tacked on to the tearoom's more permanent structure, proper construction that was *not* falling apart because it had been built with the promise of a better job later. Eunny had made it work, keeping Song's Scrap operational with patch jobs and pique, but even sheer stubbornness only lasted so long.

Stubbornness and apathy.

"We could help you with the repairs," her Auntie Yerina had said. More than once. "Turn it into a proper shop. The town loves it."

And wasn't that just the problem. The community had embraced her ramshackle café far more than Eunny could've ever hoped. She loved it, too, sort of. The idea of it. Of having a place where she would only have to fix things, never people, and with her own two, mundane hands. While she took paying work, she also opened the shop a few days a week for communal mending gatherings, and they had taken on a life of their own. Not that Eunny had been able to hold any open craft hours lately. She couldn't make the space or provide accommodation that was halfway decent, and she balked at fixing the café, making it "proper." Real. Like a place where she could belong, doing something she loved. As if she deserved either.

Shouldering open the loft's door, Eunny snagged a towel on the way to her desk, blotting the moisture from her dark hair. Thunder rumbled in the distance, the noise competing with the pounding rain on the roof. Eunny dropped into her chair, elbows going to the desktop as she sighed, rubbing her temples. Her gaze drifted along the scuffed wood, traveling down until it came to rest on the bottom drawer. With slow, reluctant movements, she dragged it open. Tucked away at the back was her old apothecarist toolkit. She pulled it out and hefted the familiar weight of it in her palm, fingers caressing the well-worn leather all creased and scuffed from what had once been frequent use. The material wasn't as flexible anymore, dried out after years of being stored away, no longer regularly handled and conditioned.

Eunny set it on the desktop, undoing the one-hand tie and unrolling it with a flick of her wrist. Muscle memory carried the motion where her conscious mind forgot. She ignored the tools that remained in the pockets of the wrap. Her variety of tweezers and any useful ingredients had long since been pressed into service at the café; she didn't need the array of scoops or cutting implements or specimen jars. She had no need to come up and look at this relic from her past with any regularity.

It had been so easy once, to feel the soft current of her magic coursing through her hands. Had hardly taken any thought to call light into her fingers, drawing from the tiny well at her center that was the source of her magic. Given the current downpour, with the rain so prevalent that even the air inside the loft felt vaguely damp, the circumstances were eerily familiar. It made the memory of magic itch along her palms.

Eunny shook her head, scattering raindrops everywhere. Not that it did much good, as more rain fell in her eyes. The tents were in ruins, the scent of smoke battling against the elements as it filtered through the air. At least the rain kept the delegation's camp from going up in flames.

The chaos began to settle as the Sentinels quelled the last of the Eyllics' desperate defense. The Eyllics who hadn't died by an arrow or blade ensured their end through other means, for apparently death was preferable to capture. Eunny's stomach tried to heave at the memory of what it had felt like trying to save one of them. Eyllic or not, enemy of the Valley—enemy of all the Empyrean Territories, for that matter—or not, Eunny was a mender first. She'd taken an oath that transcended nationality. But the empire across the sea was a master of poison, and its work was fast when needed. The oily, bitter feel of it to her magic still clung to the edges of her mind even as she reached to heal her dozenth patient. Maybe it was for the best the Eyllics weren't her problem. Unethical as the thought was, Eunny was exhausted. She was an apothecary by trade, not a practitioner of direct mending. Patching up the various wounded Sentinels and trade delegation members had her inner sphere of magic feeling dangerously low.

"Who's next?" she mumbled, eyes closing in a long blink. Her brain felt heavy, sluggish.

"I— It's okay. I'm fine, it's barely a scratch."

She looked up to see Ollas Nevin clasping a bloodied bandage around his arm. Rain had flattened his brown curls against his head, hiding a gash near his temple. She'd have missed it if the trail of red against his pale skin didn't give it away.

"Come on," she said with a weary wave of her hand. When he hesitated, she glared at him. "Get over here, Nev." An upside to

having known Ollas since they were kids: Eunny didn't need to find the energy for things like patience and professionalism.

His head wound wasn't bad, just prone to bleeding with all the rain. The slice across his arm was worse. Eunny didn't have the energy to shush Ollas's babble as she placed trembling fingers on the blood-soaked gauze pad already slapped across the wound. A dull roar began in her ears, gradually growing louder in time with her heartbeat. Ollas was the last one. She only needed to glue him back together enough to hold for just a little bit. Just long enough for her to take a nap. Then she could brew some fortifying tea, keep everyone in good shape for the trek back to... to wherever they were going. Gods, she was tired.

Ollas was talking again, voice low, hesitant. Annoyed, Eunny shook her head. He sounded so far away, and the roar in her ears wasn't dull at all anymore but a blare of incoherent noise.

Something brushed against her magic. She blinked, reflexively pushing it away, but her control was slipping, ripples coursing up her arm as sparks emanated from her fingertips. The pulling sensation intensified, tangling Eunny's threads of arcane, the pressure building until they yanked free of her. She tried to claw back control, but she was so tired. Spent. Couldn't regain control as magic was dragged from her skin and onto Ollas. Her golden light moved of its own accord as it spilled over his arm and onto his chest, sinking into him and disappearing.

Ollas screamed. He went rigid beneath her touch as his muscles seized. As abruptly as the fit had begun, his body relaxed, sagged, and in her mind's eye, Eunny felt miniscule bubbles of magic bursting beneath her fingers. His body twitched with each one, as if it stung his flesh the same way each pop seared in her head. Wisps of golden light rose from Ollas's body, turned gray like smoke, and drifted back down until he was covered in tiny motes of ash.

～

Eunny blinked away the memory. The nails of one hand had left dark crescents in her light brown palm. She forced her shaking hands flat against the desk. All was quiet now. Silent. She didn't reach for her magic. Didn't listen. Didn't try. She'd grown used to the absence. She was relieved by it, for it meant magic was dead to her.

The bell beside her desk rang, signaling the opening of the repair café's front door. Eunny jerked from her wavering thoughts, stuffing the toolkit back into the desk drawer.

"I'm here, I'm here!" She hurried down the loft's steps, cursing herself for getting lost in useless memories.

"Sorry, I don't have the whole—"

She stopped in the middle of the café's front room.

Ollas Nevin, the Homegrown Hero, darling of Sylvan, the man Eunny had broken with her wayward magic, stood at her door.

Chapter Two

OLLAS PAUSED OUTSIDE of Song's Scrap so he could shake the accumulated rainwater from his cloak's hood. In his thirty years of Valley living, he'd become well-acquainted with the region's penchant for liquid sunshine, but this was excessive even for a born-and-raised Sylvan boy. The waxed leather of his boots, imbued with magic for extra waterproofing, was starting to fail. Ollas made a mental note to swing by the Sylveren University's student-run mercantile to pick up some more shoe wax.

He peered through the window to survey the main room. Empty, though it was hard to tell with all the clutter. "Hello?" he called over the jingle of a bell attached to the door. "Eunny?"

Ollas walked to the counter to wait. One of the lamps outside the front door flickered, the illumination charm worked into the glass losing its personal battle with the rain. Maybe Gransen hadn't been exaggerating about the state of the repair café. Ollas's roommate was something of the de facto manager to the place and had gotten himself temporarily banished for bickering with Eunny one time too many about the deteriorating conditions. So Ollas had volunteered to retrieve the repair order for the Grove, the university's earth magic wing.

That it provided him an opportunity to speak with Eunny in relative privacy was purely coincidental. A nice perk. Gransen hadn't really been fooled, but he'd let Ollas trot off without comment.

For a moment, Ollas let his eyes close as he took a steadying breath. Something hummed beneath his skin, a soft little buzz, so faint he had to look for it to notice most of the time. It had been growing ever since he'd come back to the Valley at the beginning of summer. It wasn't unpleasant, but it was strange. Perhaps the feeling was commonplace for those with a strong affinity for the arcane. But for someone who barely had enough magic to be considered above a mundane, it stood out. Maybe the feeling wasn't related to magic at all but lingering stress? He'd decided to resume his role as a horticulture professor at Sylveren University instead of pursuing more graduate work. It was a choice he didn't regret, but timing meant he'd been rushing around for the last month, making all his final arrangements. The fall term was only a couple weeks away and promised to keep him busy with an Initiate One core class and joint-teaching an upper-level elective with his mentor.

Finally, Ollas had stability, a chance to stay in one place instead of shuttling back and forth every few months. And it meant he'd have time to reconnect with friends here in town. With one, in particular. Make amends, if necessary. Because he wanted Eunny Song to be able to say his name and not automatically think of the worst day of her life. He wanted—needed—her forgiveness for his part in it. For the sake of a friendship gone brittle at the edges. He'd run off and hoped being away for the last six years with the Valley's mountains between them would smooth the roughness from their interactions. The debacle at the Mighty Leaf's summer solstice party two months ago had proved that time and distance was just wishful thinking.

"I'm here, I'm here!" The sound of boots thumping down the stairs preceded the back door of the café opening and Eunny rushing in. "Sorry, I don't have the whole—"

She stopped a few paces from the counter, eyes widening as she took in his drippy appearance.

"Hi." Ollas's hand twitched with a feeble wave. "I'm here for the Grove's order?"

"Oh, right, yeah. It's over here. Sorry for the mess." Eunny motioned for him to follow her to a different area of the café.

Ollas trailed after her, nerves making his hands twitch. It was strange yet comforting how Eunny didn't acknowledge the passage of time. Whether it was mere days or upwards of six months, whenever he'd made it back to town during his Adept Two graduate studies and their paths crossed, she'd carried on as if there'd never been a break. Perhaps it shouldn't have struck him as odd, seeing as they'd known each other since they were kids, back when she'd only visited her aunt for the summers. Absences were the norm for them. And Ollas, he was pretty sure he'd been in some kind of love with her since his tweens. A feeling that couldn't be mutual, not with the way she froze upon seeing him—just for a moment, and then she was back to her usual breezy self. If only he could pretend at normalcy half so well.

Eunny reached for a box of repaired items and lifted it onto the nearest tabletop. "My apologies to the Grove folks. I'll finish the rest of the order as quick as I can."

"It's no trouble. Let me help." Ollas came forward, eyes meeting hers for the space of a breath before he flushed and looked at the box instead.

"I got it, Nev." Eunny elbowed him, an exasperated laugh taking the bite out of her words. "Could you grab the work order there?" She nodded with her chin toward a paper, one of many, on the end of the counter.

Ollas scanned the offerings, careful to pull back his wet sleeve. He held up a page, bringing it over at Eunny's nod.

"I think I've marked what's done and what's still pending, but let me check again before you leave," Eunny said as she started pulling out the completed items.

Same old Eunny. Moving on as if nothing had happened. As if she'd seen him yesterday, not back at the start of summer. Except for that moment when she'd first realized it was him at the door. That pause, the indecision. Because they could act like everything was fine, but they both remembered. Not just the summer solstice party and some nosy tourists, but the cause of said prying curiosity. The failed trade delegation that had seen Eunny held captive. The messy rescue. Eunny's magic, its featherlight touch that he barely remembered. And then...everything that had come after.

Ollas never wanted to become one of the people who badgered her about losing her magic, but when it came to *them,* that, he could try to fix.

"I never got to—"

"Listen, about what I—"

They both stopped, stared at each other. Waited a beat, then started to speak again at the same time.

Eunny put out her hand to stop him. "Pause. Let me say this. About the summer release at the Mighty Leaf. I owe you an apology."

Ollas clamped his lips together, holding back the words burning on his tongue. *You don't owe me anything. Those guys—I should've shut them up. My fault, not yours. It's no one's fucking business what happened that day.*

Eunny grimaced, a hint of pink tingeing her golden-brown skin. Eunny. Blushing. At him. "I said some—"

She was cut off. The loud groan of breaking wood split the air. The floor beneath their feet was shifting, *vibrating,* as the walls and roof shook. Eunny dropped the tray she was holding, stumbling back a step before Ollas caught her by the arm. He grabbed the countertop for support as horrid sounds of tearing, sliding, and crumpling filled his ears. The whole building shuddered.

Gods all break. He'd heard of such land shakes, but those disasters didn't occur in the Valley. On the southern coast, perhaps, but not here. He'd seen landslides during his studies in the mountains, and the Valley had some floods. But what did one do when the building threatened to tumble around you?

Get out.

He didn't think beyond that simple imperative. He slung an arm around Eunny's middle and heaved them both toward the back door. Their exit was marred by the wall buckling, displacing the furnishings below. Something long and firm struck him. A plank, maybe? A stool? Whatever it was, it had much less give than the back of his legs.

As it knocked him down, pain lanced across his shoulder, his side, above one of his knees, then bloomed into something more as he managed to stagger upright and drag Eunny into the tiny rear courtyard. A rush of air licked their backs as the ceiling caved in, a shower of wood and pieces of cheap shingle raining to the ground.

As abruptly as it had started, the shaking stopped. The noise continued, crashes echoing off the courtyard stones before fading.

The corner of the loft had collapsed near the front door, twisting the roof to let in the rain. Almost neatly down the middle, Song's Scrap had fallen into a heap. The temporary construction, weakened by the Valley's unrelenting rain and numerous spots badly in need of repairs, had finally lost its fight to remain standing. Not a land shake at all, then; only time and rot.

Where the café had been attached to the Mighty Leaf, the damaged wall and the stairway to the loft had pulled away, half of it now hanging askew.

"Oh, gods all...Fuck," Eunny said, one hand going to her mouth.

The beaten metal sign announcing "Song's Scrap" fell as if in slow motion, one end breaking from its hanger to wobble at a sharp angle. It swung back and forth, the metallic creaking loud in the eerie silence of the collapsed building.

With his adrenaline already retreating beneath the fire spreading across his body, Ollas groaned. "Are you—Are you hurt?"

"I-I don't know. What just...?" Eunny turned to him, her eyes widening. "Oh, shit, Nev, *you're* hurt!"

Her hand twitched, as if the response was automatic even after so much time. She reached toward his wound without thinking, because that's what menders did, right? If there was pain around, it was their imperative to ease it, no matter the personal cost.

Ollas wouldn't let her make that mistake again. Wouldn't encourage it.

"Don't." His hand closed over hers, nudging it away. "It's not—"

Eunny stared at him, brown eyes wide and intent, yet she seemed to be looking through him rather than at him. Remembering a moment so similar despite the difference in time. She blinked, gaze dropping to where his hand guided her away from his leg.

"Oh." Eunny recoiled. Just as she had six years ago. "Oh, of course. I... Ollas, gods. I'm sorry. Old habits."

Ollas bit back a curse and made a half-hearted motion toward her, his fingers hesitating in the air as she flinched away. "Eunny, it's not—"

A dark, choked laugh escaped her as she held up her palms. "Don't worry, I lost it, remember? You're safe from me."

"Eunny?" Her aunt's voice cut through the air, a note of panic turning it shrill.

"Back here! We need help." Eunny helped Ollas to ease his legs straight along the ground. He chanced a look down and grimaced; a tear along one trouser leg showed pale skin marred with more red. His sleeve was wet, sodden in a way that couldn't be blamed on the rain. And it hurt, Earthen take him, everything hurt ever more as awareness trickled in.

Eunny's aunt, Yerina Song-Burl, and several patrons of the Mighty Leaf rushed toward them, alarm on everyone's faces. As they bustled around him, Eunny faded into the background, and whatever hope Ollas had had at conveying his true intentions was lost.

Someone brushed against the sign for Song's Scrap as they passed. The motion caught Ollas's eye as his surroundings took on a fuzzy quality. It swayed back and forth, the hanger sagging downward. With a final snap, the sign broke free and crashed to the ground.

Chapter Three

"Absolutely not," Eunny said, ignoring the wood samples Gransen Mast tried to show her.

"Just look at them. This is a real opportunity here!" Gransen said, his tone between wheedling and exasperated.

He'd first appeared at Song's Scrap three years ago, freshly graduated from his Initiate levels and drawn in by a small tool repair demonstration being put on by a local woodworker. He was a Graelynd expatriate like Eunny, but that was where their similarities ended. He was short, stocky, with a mop of mouse-brown hair and a perpetual goofy smile. After that first repair workshop, Gransen had kept coming back, often without anything in need of repair himself. He'd just *stayed*. Considered himself her unofficial assistant. Self-proclaimed manager of Song's Scrap.

And he was taking the collapse of the café hard. Most days, Eunny appreciated his enthusiasm, but the day after the self-destruction of her home and business? No. She needed a break from his endless buzzing of ways to rebuild the shop. She hadn't even managed to get any useful information on Ollas's condition despite Gransen being his roommate, aside from a blithe, "Who do you think booted me out of the room and refused my budding skills as a nursemaid? Olly's fine."

A voice hailed her from the café's door—what was left of it. She turned to see one of her best friends, Zhenya Lee. The studious inkmaker waded through the rubble, a heap of burlap sacks from the tearoom in her arms.

"Where should I start?" Zhenya asked.

"Cabinets by the stack cutter? You'll know better than me if anything can be saved." Eunny waved toward the ancient cutting blade she'd managed to cram into a corner of the rear wall. The tool itself could probably have survived a dozen cave-ins, but the crate shelves Eunny had stacked together for holding excess bookbinding supplies, not so much. Bits of cord and ribbon in a variety of colors were nothing but tangled snarls amidst smashed glue pots and folding tools. Paper of both decorative and utilitarian sorts hadn't been cleaned up from the floor so much as swept, or shoved, into piles.

Zhenya wilted a bit at the sight but rallied with a brave smile. "I'll see what I can do."

"I'll be right there." Eunny turned to Gransen, who was sliding what looked disturbingly like fabric swatches into his bag. "Granse, what are you—"

"You're busy, and I have reading to catch up on. I'll just look through all these and bring you a short list later."

"Why do you need— Are those for *curtains?* We don't even have windows—"

"Don't worry, I'll handle it. Bye!" The miscreant's last word was drawn out behind him as he beat a hasty retreat from the shop.

Scrubbing a hand across her face, Eunny sighed and trudged over to where Zhenya picked through one of the piles. Most of it ended up in the burlap sack she'd designated for the rubbish pit. Though they were both of Hanyeok descent, instead of having dark bay-black hair Zhenya's was pearl white —a mark of her being from Deiju Island, a small island off Hanyeok's coast—and had acquired a few colorful stray threads from the bedraggled ribbons she'd rescued.

"Thanks, but you really don't have to do this." Eunny dragged one of the repair café's few surviving stools over and plopped down. "Might be a better use of everyone's time if I just threw everything away."

The Valley was showing a bit of kindness, turning the rain back to merely gray skies. But not even late summer in the Valley was the kind of weather to dry out a month's worth of rain in a single day. It did make for a more comfortable time as she logged the damages, though. A marginal amount of comfort. Really, all the log did was make it irrefutable that Song's Scrap had been a roof for junk. The scattered supplies kept for repairs might've proved useful once, but exposed to the elements and smashed to bits, they became trash just the same as the broken pieces they'd been meant to fix.

"We can salvage some." Zhenya patted another sack next to her, the gathered objects sitting atop it so small that Eunny hadn't even noticed them.

Why bother, Eunny almost said. Maybe this was a sign. She loved the town, but she'd put off turning Song's Scrap into a real building for so long. It had been something to deal with when she was ready. Once it felt deserved. Maybe the destruction was its own kind of answer.

Once they'd filled the first garbage-bound sack, Eunny lugged it to join the wreckage of the back door. As she went to grab a new sack, she noticed Zhenya had brought her satchel and left it on the front counter. "Were you working before this?"

"No. Not really," Zhenya said, her tone less than convincing. "I was just, er, getting a second opinion on my new anti-fade ink samples for the greenhouse."

Definitely working, then. Eunny had known the little white-haired inkmaker for years; some things never changed. Research and study were as much Zhenya's passions as they were her actual job, assisting the head of the botany department, Professor Rai. But a second opinion, that likely meant—

"Does that mean you've seen Ollas?" Eunny asked, wincing at how hesitant she sounded.

Eunny had known Zhenya since they were children, but with Zhenya being a few years younger, they hadn't grown from acquaintances to good friends until Eunny had moved to Sylvan six years back. And, though Zhenya was a Graelynder, too, after her Initiate levels at Sylveren University, the Valley had become her new home. Since she seemed to live between the library and the university's greenhouse complex, a friendship with Ollas had been practically inevitable.

Useful, too, with Eunny's guilt gnawing away at her. "How is he? Gransen wasn't much help when I asked."

"Just came from seeing him. He talked the menders into letting him go home already." Zhenya shook her head, a smile playing across her lips as she set some bloated paper scraps on her "save" pile. Her expression went solemn. "He's okay, but it'll be a slow process. He's worried with the term starting so soon."

"The university will give him some grace, won't they?"

"He's co-teaching a new elective with Professor Rai, doing most of the greenhouse work. He thinks he'll need to— Well, I probably shouldn't... He's just worrying." Zhenya flushed, ducking her head.

"Sorry, I didn't mean to pry," Eunny mumbled. Remorse churned in her gut. Bad enough that Ollas had gotten hurt in her damned café, trying to keep *her* safe. But now it might screw up his own work? Gods all break. Eunny Song, wrecking lives and *livelihoods*. Maybe that was a tad melodramatic, but co-teaching sounded like a big opportunity for a relatively young, low-magic-base professor like Ollas.

She glanced toward the back door, biting her lip as she recalled the way she'd reached out, unthinking. And how he'd stopped her. She remembered what had happened the last time she'd tried to heal him.

"Can't the students help out?" Eunny asked.

"Yes, but they're only in the greenhouses during lab hours, or they'll have their other classes to work on. Ollas does a lot of prep and extra work outside of the usual times. He's thorough. It's why he's such a good fit for the elective."

Zhenya started to muse aloud over the potential replacements if Ollas resigned, but Eunny's attention was split. There had to be some way she could make this right without trying to heal him again. It was an understatement to say she didn't know much about growing things. She struggled to grow weeds. Back when she did her apothecary work, she'd been unashamed to only use acquired ingredients rather than try to raise a backyard medicinal garden. But it sounded like Ollas just needed an able body.

He might already see her as the Healer Who Hurts, but she wouldn't have *Derailer of Careers* added to her list of titles.

If it meant helping Ollas keep his job, she'd tote him around on her back to water every plant in the greenhouse by hand.

The sky was starting to darken as Eunny approached the Grove, domain of the earth mages at Sylveren University. She'd been back on campus several times since the trade delegation had gone awry. The rescue. The day her magic failed. But she'd never been in the great tree, only around the greenhouses. It felt a little strange, but not uncomfortable. No flares of hostility, no surges of anger bubbling beneath her skin like she got when she was around the House of Syvrine and its healing ward.

Toward the Grove, she felt only curiosity. Maybe a bit of awe. The large maple tree soared as tall as the elementalists' towers on Sylveren University's campus, its fiery leaves imparting an autumnal feel year-round. Tiny motes of golden light twinkled throughout the foliage, lazily drifting skyward, a few sparkles bouncing off the windows as they made their journey up.

Buildings had been constructed in harmony with the massive tree, some within and others winding throughout the sturdy trunk and its lower branches. At the base of the trunk was the entrance to the Heartwood, the locus of all Grove activity. Eunny bypassed the bustle of the common room and clambered up the staircase to the residential branch of the Grove before she lost her nerve. It would be fine.

Finding the apartment Ollas and Gransen shared wasn't hard, despite Eunny never having seen it before. Gransen had no shame or sense of oversharing the whereabouts of the apartment he shared with the professor. She'd heard enough "Don't be such a prude, Eunny," and "He's not my advisor, Eunny," and "We're both Adept levels, Eunny," to no longer have a second thought about said living arrangements.

She paused outside the door, eyeing the brass nameplate marking it as *O. Nevin and G. Mast*. This might be another mistake. There was an obvious discomfort that existed between her and Ollas, even if it mostly lived beneath the surface of their long, casual friendship. Her being here, half-baked proposition in mind, had a good chance of making everything even more fraught.

But he was talking about dropping out of this special class. A collab with Professor Rai, which was a rare opportunity for younger faculty like Ollas, according to Zhenya. Her friend could get intense and hyperbolic about her work, but the only plant nerd Eunny knew to rival Zhen was Ollas. Which was probably why *they* were friends. And this was all Eunny's fault.

She had a plan, and if it was too uncomfortable for him, he could always say no.

Eunny rapped on the door.

"Hang on." Shuffling steps preceded the door opening. "Sorry, takes me—" Ollas broke off as his eyes snapped to her and went wide with recognition. Wariness.

Eunny froze mid-greeting, her brain stuttering to a halt. Ollas stood shirtless in the doorway, leaning on a cane. His torso and one arm were covered in enough bandages to almost replace a shirt. *Almost.* Fair skin dusted with freckles peeked out around the medical wraps. A hint of abs. Definition of shoulder and chest when he tensed at the sight of her, as if gathering to flee.

"Hell-o. Oh. Hi." Eunny realized she was staring, gaze roving over Ollas like he was a piece of meat despite being clad in bandages. He wasn't what one would call bulky, but she'd known he was fit from his ranger work with the Sentinels and being a garden gnome for the university. Still, this was... unexpected.

Ollas flushed.

Get a grip, Eun, what is wrong with you? *No ogling your friend who is bruised and bloodied and slow to heal because of you.* Eunny forced her mouth closed, lips pressed together in a tight smile. She renewed her small wave. "Sorry to make you get up." She gestured toward his crutch. "Got a moment?"

"Sure, of course," Ollas said faintly. Everything about him looked faint, come to think of it, and Eunny's guilty conscience couldn't decide if she hoped it was due to his recent blood loss or not. Otherwise, he was dismayed at her mere presence, which wasn't encouraging.

Eunny walked into the front room. It served triple duty as an entryway, small kitchen, and dining area, with a short hallway off to the side. A lounge along one wall had been converted into a bed, presumably to save Ollas a few more steps as he recovered. The sight caused a fresh wave of guilt to squirm around her insides, but it also imparted a shot of resolve.

Ollas lowered himself onto the edge of the bed, dragging his green Sentinels' cloak on for more cover as Eunny grabbed a chair. "Were you looking for Gransen? He went down—"

"No, I'll deal with the gremlin later," Eunny muttered, and sat, fighting the urge to jiggle her leg. "Ollas. I'm really sorry about what happened. The shop's been a mess for— If I hadn't just been standing around like a fucking knob, you wouldn't have—"

"Eunny, it isn't your fault."

"It is!" Eunny plowed on before he could protest again. "I heard about the special course you have this term, and that you're worried about it."

"Who—" Ollas started to ask, then grimaced. "Zhenya."

"She can't help herself. You know how she is about classes, you can't stop her." Eunny scoffed, but there was a lightheartedness to the sound. A smile cracked Ollas's lips in response. "Since it's my fault your position with the— *Shush*, it is! Listen, you can't lose it because of my café crashing down on you. So, I'm offering to help."

"Help?" Ollas said.

"With whatever you needed two arms and legs for," Eunny said.

"I can't ask— I appreciate it, truly, I do. But I couldn't ask you to do that," Ollas mumbled. "I'll have the students to assist with the heavy lifting."

"I'm offering. Insisting, adamantly. And if it was as simple as having them carry your stuff around during class, you wouldn't have worried about this to Zhenya." She gave him a mock stern look. "I'm not pretending to know anything about plants, but I'm guessing you work a lot more than just during class hours."

Ollas remained quiet, his gaze dropping to the edges of the blanket covering his bed.

Eunny sighed. "Can you tell me a bit more about the class? Graduate work?"

"A mix of Initiate Fours and Adept levels," Ollas said. "The Restorers are funding a grant so we can try to improve the main plants used in bioremediation efforts. Study cycles of growth and how adjustments at various stages can affect the plants. We're hoping to improve the seed stock being used in Rhell's new containment wards."

"Seeing as one of my best friends in the whole world is up there fighting the good fight, I'm on board with this plan," Eunny said.

Six years had passed since the unofficial war with Eylle had been declared over, yet the poison corrupting Rhell, the Valley's northern neighbor, remained strong as ever. Anything that helped keep Dae safe had Eunny's fervent approval. Though Dae and her lover, Ezzyn Sor'vahl, had seen recent successes in containing the poison, a true cure still remained out of reach.

"You're more on the growing end?" she asked.

He nodded. "Professor Rai's side will handle end-use with the plants and spell applications."

He explained how the plants being used for restoration efforts were finicky. The elective aimed to hybridize fast-growing plants with slower types that boasted robust ice and heat resistance. The school had received seeds from several Radiant Isles strains, along with more amendments to try, all to design and grow a new cultivar. In one academic term.

"I take it that's not much time for something like this?" Eunny said.

Ollas huffed, pinching the bridge of his nose. "It's— It's practically impossible. There are so many variables to record. We'll use probes, but they're not the same as being able to dig your fingers into the soil and observe and document from touch. We'll be making minute adjustments at every step of the process." His shifted to cradle the side of his face, a frown marring his brow. "One term isn't enough time. The successive planting, monitor the watering, make adjustments to the soil. There's so much trialing—"

"Sounds like the class really needs you, then. And"—she waved a hand at his injuries—"you need an extra set of hands, and a leg, no magic necessary. I can be that for you."

"Eunny, I can't ask—"

"*I'm offering.* At this point, I'm basically telling you. I'm doing this."

"The café—"

"Isn't going to be open for a while. I need some time, not just to clean up but to figure out what I'm going to do with it."

"Gransen can help me," Ollas said.

"Gransen has his own classes. I'm here. I'm unemployed at the moment, and I'm of able body. Let me help you out."

When it looked like Ollas would protest again, Eunny winced. A quiet sigh escaped as she shook her head, eyes meeting his for a moment before she looked down at her hands. Made loose fists before slowly releasing, palms up, fingers intertwining. Softly, she said, "Term starts soon. You'd only be ready for it if you could take healing magic."

"Eunny..." Ollas fidgeted. "It's not all on you. I was there—"

She looked at him again, the corners of her mouth lifting in a sad smile. "I'm the reason you can't anymore. We both know it."

Her magic going rogue, breaking away from her, twisting into something volatile and uncontrollable as it misfired straight into Ollas—she'd been warned of the risks in pushing beyond one's limits, same as every other mender, but she'd never experienced the consequences firsthand. A dangerous combination of ignorance and arrogance in her mid-twenties had left her convinced that reaching the dregs of her inner well would merely leave her exhausted, sapped of magic until she had a chance to rest. Maybe she'd feel like shit from overextending, sure, but she'd thought her magic would just run out, not go into freefall. Not go against the very core of what her magical affinity *was*. Not *harm* instead of *heal*.

A costly mistake. A mistake that had broken her trust in magic, in herself and whatever ability she'd thought she had. But what did trust or confidence matter in the grand scheme of things? Those were just intangible pieces of emotion that could be shoved into a little box and tossed to the back of her mind. Broken faith was nothing compared to a broken body. Damaging Ollas's ability to absorb healing magic, *that* was substantial and real and entirely her fault. It was unforgivable. So, to be the cause of him losing something else...

Eunny would not be the reason again. Not if she could do anything to prevent it.

She straightened, eyebrows lifting as she tried to lighten the mood. "It's just for a few weeks, right?" She pointed to his bandages. "I can smell the salve from here. Better than nothing, but you won't be ready by the time term starts."

"It'll be so boring for you," Ollas said, a pleading look in his eyes. "I keep long hours at the start of class, especially one like this."

"Perfect. I was a champ at all-nighters. Who needs sleep?"

"It's all repetition, and it's dirty work," he tried again.

"We're going to be starting tons of seeds, and most will probably fail, and then we'll have to restart."

"Busy work. Sign me up."

Ollas appeared torn between skepticism and something like hope.

"Great," Eunny said. "Meet tomorrow for my crash course in all things gardening?"

"At least let me get you listed as a consultant," Ollas said. "We have some room with the grant."

She was shaking her head before he finished. "Thanks, but I don't want a real commitment with the school. I'm supposed to be helping you out, not job-hunting."

"But the café—"

"Don't worry about it." She got up, flashing a quick smile. "I'll see if the housing department has something for me. It'll be easier if you're not having to send for me down in town."

Ollas reached for his cane. "I can ask at the desk."

Eunny waved him back down. "I'll use your name. Don't fret."

"If you're sure," he said dubiously.

He might be dubious, but Eunny heard the note of relief in his voice. When she grinned at him, a shy smile spread across his face in return. A real smile, not an *I'm humoring you* grimace.

After agreeing to meet another day so they could have a mini-orientation, Eunny left. It was too late for any of the administration offices to be open, but first thing tomorrow, she'd get her name on a list at housing. She wasn't thrilled at the idea of living at the school again, but a real bed sure beat Auntie Yerina's floor.

It was silly, but Eunny fought the urge to skip as she descended the stairs. Sure, guilt was still a leaden mass on her soul, but this felt like progress. A baby step in the right direction. Redistributing her mountain of atonement with a tooth-pick, perhaps, but now, she was armed for the process.

Eunny made her way toward the main road, passing by the greenhouse at the farthest edge of the Grove's complex. An overgrown patch of nondescript plants spread alongside the rear corner of the building, their long, strappy, grass-like leaves sprawling across the narrow path.

She walked by, brushing the leaves with her leg—

"Whoa!" The touch set off a flurry of twitches in her eye, making Eunny stumble sideways. In the gloom of the off-hours lighting, she missed how the stones of the path were slightly elevated above the overgrown plot. Off-balance, she tripped and fell to her knees amidst the grassy clumps.

"Gods all fucking... *break.*" She gasped as the minute spasms in her eye immediately stilled, replaced by the oddly familiar sense of restlessness that had plagued her all summer. The pulling sensation revived, emanating from her center. From the little sphere next to her heart, the inner well where her magic used to dwell.

Except, not *used to.*

"Oh, shit," she moaned. "No, no, no."

Eunny could declare magic was dead to her—and mean it—but saying it was so and *making* it so, well... With great, grudging reluctance, she'd have to admit those weren't the same thing. Six years ago, magic had betrayed her. In the face of it, Eunny had willfully left the idea of her magic behind, excised all trace of it from her mental being as best she could. But conflating disuse and death, that was just her own wishful thinking.

The grass-like leaves clung to her hands. When she tried to shake free, something *pulled* at her. The horrible sensation of her magic being dragged from beneath her skin, just like the day she'd lost control. That same feeling of slipping, careening toward a crash. And that brief moment of icy clarity right before impact, knowing she couldn't stop.

Eunny ripped her hand back and staggered onto the path. A trail of golden sparks rippled in her wake and fell to the mounds of grass. The sparks didn't wink out so much as sink into the leaves, absorbed like water into blotting paper.

"What— What the...?" Eunny stared at her hands, then the plants, head whipping back and forth. Her eye was calm, the imperceptible feelings of restlessness, of being called to, gone quiet. Eunny didn't dare look inward at the hole that was supposed to be the only remnant of her magic.

Panic rose in her throat as the realization of what had happened struck. She looked around. No witnesses. Her gaze landed on the clumps of grass sitting there all benign and giving the impression of just being bland foliage. Eunny hurried away, not stopping until she reached the campus's main courtyard. Only then did she pause and glance back in the direction of the greenhouse complex. The distance and the darkness didn't matter—the image of the grassy clumps sitting there, as if they were no more than bland foliage, immediately came to Eunny's mind.

"Never again." She spat on the ground. "You're not getting shit from me."

Chapter Four

"I'm confused," Gransen said. "Shouldn't your new valet be doing this part?"

"Don't call her that," Ollas muttered, glancing up and down the hall, but Eunny was nowhere in sight.

Which was to be expected, seeing as they hadn't planned on meeting to familiarize her with the greenhouse complex until later in the afternoon. No reason to expect to find her in the university administration building.

"I thought the whole point of her becoming your personal aide was to provide, you know, aid." Gransen lifted Ollas's bag of books and amendment samples in one hand, and the stack of papers that hadn't fit amongst them in the other.

"Only once classes start." Ollas reached for the papers destined for turn-in at the registrar's desk. "I *said* I could manage."

Gransen skipped out of reach. "Don't be ridiculous. You're broken. What kind of person would make his critically injured best friend haul his shattered—"

Ollas poked Gransen in the shin with his cane. "There'll be a statue of you in the courtyard any day now, I'm sure."

Gransen heaved a dramatic sigh. "I wish they wouldn't. Sculptors never get my hair right."

Ollas continued down the hall, but Gransen easily kept pace with his limp.

"Give me the truth, though. Why are you being so weird about this?" Gransen asked. "It's ideal. You, injured, and Eunny nursing you back—"

"Me being injured is your version of ideal?"

"Are we really going to pretend that this isn't the perfect opportunity?"

"For?" Ollas said, voice stubbornly neutral.

Gransen tipped his head back and made an exasperated noise. "You save her life. She saves your job. You're hurt, she's helping. You're going to be in the greenhouse. A lot. *Alone.*" He gave Ollas a sidelong look. "Are you going to make me say it? This is your chance, Olly."

"We... you know, friends. And I feel bad about it."

"Why? The woman you're *pining* over just volunteered to be your personal helper while you recover—a deal you accepted. But you're sulking and peeking around every corner like you're afraid we'll run into her. Explain to me how that works out."

"I didn't ask— She felt bad and I—" Ollas floundered for a response. For words that could explain the conflicting emotions roiling in his chest. Because, though Ollas wouldn't admit it aloud, Gransen wasn't entirely wrong. Eunny's offer, and what it entailed, it was the kind of opportunity Ollas had been hoping for ever since he'd accepted the teaching job at Sylveren. A chance to be back in town with a level of permanence. To make amends for past wrongs. The collapse of the café was an unwanted wrinkle in those plans.

"She only offered because she feels bad. Responsible," Ollas said with a grimace. "Not just the café, but for, you know. Before. I feel like I'm taking advantage of her guilt."

Not to mention his own shame. Her magic had backfired, but he'd been responsible for the ordeal, too. Earned that damned nickname, the Homegrown Hero, because he'd been the one to lead his Sentinels group to the camp where the trade delegation was being held captive. Never mind that none of them had known the delegation had gone so badly, that the Eyllics had gone back on their word and refused to let anyone leave the camp until a favorable deal was struck. Or that Ollas had thought he was simply following the trail of poachers and had found their hidden cache.

It had been chaos, those moments of finding out the cache was really the delegation's camp. Ollas remembered digging through the supply crates, so naïve in his curiosity about the foreign plants and seeds he'd found, thinking it was just the spoils of illegal harvesting. Remembered being interrupted by the sounds of screams and fighting. Recalled running off to join the chaos, to help, for whatever he was worth. Ollas was a decent enough ranger, but the Sentinels had let him stay on more for his forestry knowledge than any martial skill.

Perhaps none of that was blameworthy. But he'd seen how exhausted Eunny was after hours of healing, applying magic in a way she wasn't properly trained for. He should've refused when she offered to mend him, too. His wounds could've waited until they made it to the Sentinels' nearest outpost. But he'd wanted to feel her touch. Her magic. When else would he ever get the chance? When the opportunity presented itself, he indulged. What had happened after—his inability to heal, having to stop active patrolling with the Sentinels because such lack was a liability—it was his penance for being weak. Horrible, yes, but brought upon himself.

Gransen watched Ollas's face, solemnity replacing his usual joviality. "It's understandable," he said slowly, "why she'd feel that way, given what happened. But things are good between you, right? You seem fine, from what I've seen."

The safe, mild interactions that were inevitable in a town the size of Sylvan. Inescapable, when his mother and her aunt were so close. And brief, for Ollas had spent so much time up in the mountains for his Adept Two studies. It was easy to stay friendly when the relationship never went deeper than the surface. But go down a layer or two?

You're safe from me.

Eunny's bitter words rang in his head. The lingering spot of tension that was still alive between them, so quickly recalled, was his to fix. Until then, he didn't deserve her friendliness, let alone anything resembling affection.

"Are you at all"—Gransen made a questioning motion with his hands—"maybe a taddy bit resentful still about—"

"No." The emphatic decisiveness of the word took Ollas by surprise, but in an affirming way. He meant it. Good to know his subconscious was on board. "No, not at all. It was my— It was bad luck, is all. Who could've known?"

"Glad that's settled." Gransen said, a mischievous glint in his eye. "I'll ask her—"

"Don't."

"—all subtle-like. You'll see." Gransen gave a dismissive flutter of his fingers as Ollas tried to protest. "We have a rapport. It's how I got to be manager of the café."

"She calls you the café gremlin."

"It's a term of endearment."

"Isn't the reason I was the one picking up the order because you got yourself banned?"

"And I was right about the condition of the place, wasn't I?" Gransen smirked. "It'll be fine. I've got your back."

"Don't make things weird for me, please, Granse," Ollas

said. Then, in a low mutter, "I'm not really the type of guy she's interested in, anyway."

"Earthen take you if you were," Gransen said. "Short-lived flings with Renstownies. Aim higher, Olly, darling."

Hiding a smile, Ollas moved stiffly down the hall. At least his injuries were on opposite sides, and he could manage a cane. Once he'd dropped a few forms off with Administration for the Initiate One Basics of Arcane Soil Development class, then he could sit for a minute. Despite his protesting, he would've been in a bad way if not for Eunny's offer to help with his greenhouse duties. Just getting from his apartment in the Grove to the classrooms was going to be a chore.

"What do you mean, 'unavailable?'" Eunny's familiar voice carried around the corner. "I was just here this morning and—"

A softer voice interrupted Eunny, too low for Ollas to hear the words. Eunny's answering sigh was enough of a hint that whatever had been said earlier in the day no longer applied.

"Do you have anything else available? Preferably not in—"

Ollas and Gransen walked around the corner in time to hear the housing clerk say, "The prospective student rooms in the House of Syvrine are clear."

Eunny's eyes closed in a long blink, reticence writ large across her face.

"What happened?" Ollas asked.

"Nev. Gremlin," Eunny said by way of greeting. "I'm cursed."

Ollas cast a questioning glance at Gransen, who shrugged.

"The section in Belle Complex for overflow faculty is under emergency construction. Initiate Fours too excited for the start of their last year." The clerk shrugged. "All of our other options are full in the meantime. The best I can do today is the prospective students' rooms."

Eunny shook her head, mouth twisting with a wry grimace.

"Already paid my dues. Prospies are in the thick of it." She snorted, a touch of fond humor replacing her disdain. At Ollas's blank look, she added, "Get the prospies sloshed, then surround them with a bunch of baby mages learning body magic in earnest for the first time, all puffed up thinking they know how to mix up a hangover remedy. It's not pretty."

The clerk disguised what Ollas was pretty sure was a laugh with a delicate cough. "I'll put you on the waitlist."

Eunny bobbed her head in thanks.

They stepped away from the desk to make space for the next person in line. Gransen nudged Ollas. Then nudged him again when Ollas didn't react. "What?"

"I have an idea," Gransen said.

"No." The word was out of Eunny's mouth before he'd finished talking. "Sorry, Granse. Force of habit. You were saying?"

"We've got space, right, Olly?"

"Uh." An odd blend of horror and hope surged within him as Ollas gleaned his friend's intent. "Yes?"

Eunny's head whipped toward him, a questioning look in her eyes. Brown eyes were the most beautiful, he'd always thought, and Eunny's above all others. They were also scary as they narrowed in his direction. But then her lips twitched.

"Going to milk those injuries for all they're worth?" Her attempt at sounding wry failed when she gave a cackle. "Want me to stick around?"

Yes, always. Not that he could ever say as much.

"We have the adjoining room free," Gransen said. "I mean, there's all your old teaching stuff in there, but we can shove that to the side." He handed Ollas's bag to Eunny. "I've got to go. Ollas can give you the details."

He waved, his grin suspiciously large as he tried to convey something to Ollas, only Ollas was too dazed at the sudden turn of events to understand. A swooping sensation looped through him. Made his knees go weak, had him gripping his cane with renewed strength.

Eunny noticed. "Steady on, there. You sure you're up for our greenhouse thing?"

"I was—" He could drop the papers off later. "Yea. I think I just need to sit for a second."

They made their way outside. Ollas followed her to the university's large courtyard, pausing where the road diverged. Several paths split off to the different magic regions while one carried on straight to the main gate and back down to Sylvan. Ollas lowered himself onto one of the benches scattered around the courtyard, stretching out his aching leg. People filtered past all around them, students and university staff alike. The campus had the charged atmosphere that always preceded the start of fall term, an excitement and sense of freshness unique to this time of year. Spring term had its own energy, but it didn't quite match the anticipation that came from a summer off. A young woman, who Ollas recognized from the Initiate One Crop Planning Basics course he'd taught a few years ago, twirled around one of the decorative statuaries, singing out, "Home!" A few more of his previous students followed, waving and murmuring greetings of "Hi, Professor Nevin."

Ollas waved. The ball of tension that had been building in him lessened some, a soft smile spreading across his face. He'd enjoyed his Adept Two research up in the mountains, but had missed being able to teach with regularity.

"Feeling's mutual, isn't it?" Eunny murmured.

He glanced at her. She wasn't looking at him, her face upturned to the gray sky as clouds sped across the Valley. It was easier to regard her this way. In profile, her sharp gaze aimed at something else. It gave him a quiet moment to simply look at her. Note a flicker of concern on her face. Eunny nibbled at her lower lip, a sense of weariness creeping in that she'd hidden before.

In that unguarded moment, Eunny looked vulnerable. It drove his lingering doubts and insecurities aside as he was overwhelmed by a desire to fix whatever troubled her. To save her, however he was able. It was a compulsion, sudden and hot in his chest, a *need* to see her laugh again, carefree and happy. The Eunny Song he'd always known, until one moment of stupid, selfish weakness had taken a part of her away.

She tilted her head to the side, caught him looking. The seriousness vanished, replaced by a casually raised eyebrow. "What?"

The rush of courage ebbed, leaving a sense of bitter regret in its wake. Eunny didn't need protecting, least of all from him.

"Nothing."

She sighed. "Tell Gransen thanks, but I'm fine. It should only take you a few weeks to be mended enough. I can walk up—"

"You should take it. The room," Ollas said softly.

"Oh?" A smile played at the edges of her mouth. "Convince me."

Butterflies tickled his belly. Ollas forced himself to look toward the Grove's giant tree lest he read into her smile. "It's the Grove. The room Gransen mentioned was supposed to be a single, but something happened during construction. It's connected to our unit now."

"What's it like living there?" she asked. "The Grove. Aside from when I stormed your place, I've never been in the residential areas."

"Pretty quiet. Doesn't have any dedicated prospective student housing, and only Initiate Fours get room options. Everyone else is Adept levels or higher." Her interest was piqued, expression thoughtful. He pressed on, grasping for what he loved most about the Grove. "There's always something going on in the Heartwood. People are cooking or baking with stuff they're growing for class or a project, and they always have extra."

"That does sound nice," Eunny admitted. "A lot better than my aunt's floor."

"Think about it, please," he said, eyes cast downward. "You're offering to do this because of me—"

"Eunny! Ollas!"

They turned in unison to see Zhenya hurrying toward them. "Professor Saren—I mean, Professor Rai—wants to meet about the elective. Word just came in from the Restorers' rep about an amendment."

"Take a breath, Zhen," Eunny said as the younger woman came to a stop in front of them and doubled over, hands on her knees. "The Restorers, eh?"

The Restorers of the Alliance was a new organization, formed back at the end of spring, bringing together people from all the Alliance of Empyrean Territories to pool resources in the name of environmental restoration. Though their purview would extend to ecological damage in any region, the bulk of the organization's focus centered in the kingdom of Rhell. Curing the cursed poison that had been relentlessly making its way toward the kingdom's magical wellspring had proven impossible so far, but hope remained. Research projects carried out by Eunny's best friend Anadae Helm and her partner Ezzyn Sor'vahl had made the first breakthrough in halting the blight's spread. Containment, not a cure, but it was the first real stride made in the six years since the unofficial Eyllic War had been declared over.

Unsurprising, then, that the Restorers would make forays into Sylveren University itself; the school had been instrumental in Anadae and Ezzyn's success. Ollas knew he was biased, but Sylveren had the best professors this side of the Great Sea. It lured the brightest minds in the world, both nonmagical and arcane-born, to carry out their research. If they were going to make claims about being at the forefront of environmental restoration, there was no better institution for the Restorers to partner with than the school.

So, a last-minute changeup in curriculum? Ollas didn't know if that boded well or ill.

"He said urgent," Zhenya said with an emphatic gesture.

Ollas glanced at Eunny, a question in his eyes.

"I'm nosy." She wrapped the edges of her cloak around her as the wind picked up. "I want to hear what the Restorers have to say."

Chapter Five

Eunny knew she wasn't part of the magical community anymore, not really. She lived in Sylvan, but she wouldn't let herself feel like she *belonged*. Like it was a place and a life that could still be hers. The Healer Who Hurts didn't deserve that, regardless of who her auntie was. Eunny had lost the right to feel at home, the *will* for it. She didn't want it back...

Most days, she didn't want that old life back. Didn't miss it, because she didn't let herself think about it, about how her current stasis with a crumbly repair shop wasn't at all what she'd pictured. Yet here she was, following the others back to the Grove, her head still spinning with Ollas's... offer.

She couldn't figure him out. He'd been awkward yet earnest at the repair café. Even more so when she'd come to pitch her idea of helping him out during his recovery. But it wasn't the easy, casual camaraderie she remembered from their childhood, or the fleeting encounters when they'd chanced upon each other around town as adults.

Ollas walked slightly ahead of her, limping along well enough with his cane. He chatted amiably with Zhenya. Something about worms and mash and tea, which Eunny hoped to the gods was a garden thing and not something she'd be asked to weigh in on. Topic aside, it didn't escape her notice that Ollas had no trouble conversing with Zhenya. Shared a laugh, nodding along when Zhen got going about her latest ink experiment. Conversation between them flowed in a way that had something disturbingly like envy settling in Eunny's gut. Which was ridiculous; she knew they were friends—they were friends with *her!*—and had more in common with each other than with Eunny. Sweet, bookish nerds. But Ollas even murmured a few greetings to fellow grovetenders as they made their way to the branch where the faculty offices were housed. There was an easy confidence about him on campus that he didn't share when it was just them.

Eunny suppressed a sigh. Maybe it'd be better to decline his housing offer with as much grace as she could muster.

Professor Saren Rai was waiting for them in his office. Eunny had met Zhenya's advisor-slash-mentor-slash-boss several times since her own Initiate years and had heard about him many times over. Of Hanyeok descent like Eunny and Zhenya, his jet-colored hair had the beginnings of gray streaks. He appeared in his late forties—maybe early fifties; hard to tell after a certain point—and stood around six feet, long of frame with a slight hunch to the shoulders and bump of a belly. That, coupled with an underlying paleness to his light brown skin, betrayed the fact that he spent most of his time indoors, though his pallor was counteracted by colorful ink stains on his fingers. Both Zhenya and her mentor sported an aggressive violet today, the hue fading to pink at the edges.

Rai looked up from the papers scattered across his desk. "Ah, Miss Lee, you found them. Ollas," he said, nodding to greet him, before landing on Eunny. "Hello, Miss Song."

Eunny blinked with surprise that the head of the botany

department knew who she was, but apparently one of her friends had already made her proposed role known.

"The Restorers want to change something about the elective?" Ollas said as they all took seats.

Rai regarded them, expression grave. "The rate of illness stemming from poison exposure in Rhell is increasing. The Restorers ask that, in addition to the current bioremediation work, the elective run trials on an additional healing cultivar to improve its hardiness. Even better if we can somehow combine the two."

Both Zhenya and Ollas made sounds of dismay.

"It's contained, isn't it?" Eunny asked before Rai had finished speaking. "In Rhell. The new ward configuration Dae— I thought the containment measures were working."

"They are, as far as anyone in the Rhellian government or with the Restorers have said." Rai made a soothing gesture. "However, no one could've anticipated how it would react in containment. No one has died, to be clear."

As if death was the worst that could happen to a body.

"But?" she pressed.

"More are falling ill." Rai sighed. "Availability of arable land in the region has been tumultuous for quite some time, so any progress we make toward improved efficiency will be put to use."

Ollas cleared his throat, continuing in a low tone, "The menders can't help?"

"Certainly, but serious afflictions? No more than they have since the beginning with this poison. These newer ailments are less entrenched, but it pulls magic and energy away from where it's needed." Rai glanced at all three of them, gaze lingering on Eunny. "I trust that you will keep this in confidence?"

A soft chorus of assurances led him to give a tired nod in acknowledgement. "The students will recognize the benefits of the materials we're working with, but this development in the containment zones isn't to be made public."

"I have a lighter courseload this term already, so I'll do all I can." Ollas's brow furrowed. "I've got some ideas for adjusting the lectures and lab approach."

They began discussing an amendment to the syllabus, with Zhenya interjecting details of Rai's other commitments as they applied. It wasn't lost on Eunny how self-assured Ollas was when it came to his teaching duties. A stark contrast when compared to their own interactions.

Ollas was naturally kind of shy and quiet, but they'd been friends. *Were* friends. The delegation-turned-kidnapping-turned-rescue had changed things, of course it had. Eunny knew it. And now, after Song's Scrap collapsing, things were even more fraught. Like he'd retreated into his shell, wary of her even though the glimmers of that old friendship came through. Or was she just imagining it, so determined not to let her fucked-up break with magic control her that she couldn't see how their friendship had fractured? Or maybe she'd always assumed it was more solid a friendship than reality had proved it to be.

But then, Ollas wouldn't offer up his spare room if he didn't want her around. Would he?

Quietly, Eunny let her gaze linger on him as the three grovetenders deliberated. Even when Ollas pushed back against some of Rai or Zhenya's suggestions he didn't become loud or arrogant. Eunny didn't follow the plant jargon they all were using, but she recognized competence when she saw it. And in Ollas it was... alluring. In a way that had her tilting her head, an unspoken *huh* behind closed lips. Not unlike how she'd felt when he answered his door clad more in bandages than clothes.

Nope. Eunny gave herself a mental shake. Inappropriate

thoughts at any time, but especially now. *Get back to just being able to talk like normal people, Eun.*

She banished the image of Ollas's chest and tried to ignore his smooth confidence while in his element. It was alarmingly more difficult than she'd expected. Something to noodle over later. But as she redirected her focus to what Professor Rai had said, his grim revelations quickly consumed her. Troubles in Rhell and the containment effort, people catching sickness from fighting the poison—yet she hadn't heard a peep from Dae about any of it.

Fear wound around Eunny's heart. She'd had a letter from Dae not a week ago, and it hadn't mentioned *anything*. A gross omission Eunny would be addressing as soon as she got ahold of a pen. But why would Dae keep it a secret? No, Eunny didn't talk about her magic or lack of it anymore, but Dae knew she could speak in generalities with Eunny. She lived with magic, but not *with* magic; there was a difference. Maybe *the public* wasn't supposed to know, but Eunny wasn't the public. They were best friends. Best friends didn't keep serious shit like this from—

Oh, fuck.

If Dae was sick...

No, she couldn't be. Even if Dae was stubborn enough to be on some "I didn't want you to worry" nonsense, Ezzyn would boil the Sylvanor River in his haste to get Dae to safety in the Valley. If he hadn't sent word either, then it couldn't have touched them. Yet.

The truth of the situation was enough to make Eunny choke down a frustrated scream, drawing Ollas's attention. Concern marred his features.

Eunny shook her head. Dae was at the heart of the poison containment efforts. Eunny's conflicted feelings about being back at Sylveren and hovering at the edges of magic and the community and a semblance of what her life might've been if not for losing control in a most devastating fashion—none of it mattered. Sure, the Restorers had just added more work to an already impossible demand. This semester was about to be a great pain to all of them, including an assistant like her. But if she toddled back to the dead end that currently was the state of her repair café, she'd never hear about the evolving situation in Rhell. Not right away. But while she was around the Grove? On hand for the elective? If any more news came in from the Restorers about what was happening in Rhell, Ollas would know. Which meant Eunny could know, too. Ollas might be awkward with her, but she doubted he could lie. Not if she flat out asked. And he still got an extra pair of able hands in the deal.

"Miss Song, any input you have with regard to the mending aspects is, of course, welcome," Rai said, drawing Eunny back to the present conversation.

She cracked a weak smile. "Maybe. I never was a good hand at growing things."

Won't be around long enough to contribute anything useful, either.

"Perhaps we'll benefit from your fresh eyes," Rai said. "Would you mind if I had a word with these two? We need to discuss specifics for the course."

"No problem." Eunny stood up and glanced at Ollas. "Orient me on the greenhouse later?"

Ollas excused himself, stepping with her outside the office.

His shoulders hunched. "I can't ask you to do this. Two trials—it's going to be even more work than—"

"Again, I'm offering, not being asked. And it's decided." She gave him a light smack on the arm. "I'll be there for you for the gardening part. Will I be any good at it? Maybe, but in many ways, actually probably no. But I'll be your arms and legs, and you can direct me."

Ollas laughed softly, shoulders relaxing.

"And, if we're talking adjustments for body magic, that—" Eunny caught herself from admitting anything like a current relationship to magic. Stopped short of acknowledging it as if it was still a part of her. As if it was something welcome and useful. "Eh, I know the work," she finished instead.

"If you're sure," Ollas said slowly, but was that a note of hope she heard? Uncertainty, but in a good way.

"I am." And then, since joking with him seemed to bring back some of their old comfort with each other, Eunny gave him a sly smile. "And, I accept, by the way."

"Accept?"

"Your offer." She laughed. "We're going to be roommates, Nev."

"Oh. *Oh,* that's right. I mean, that's nice. Good." Ollas blushed, one hand coming up to cover his smile. "I'm glad."

Something warm coursed through her at his reaction.

"If we're not orientating now," she said, "then I'll head back to town and let Auntie Yerina know my plans. I'll come up tonight."

"Okay." A faint blush still shone through the stubble on Ollas's cheeks, but he met her smile with his own. "I'll find you later, then." He waved, then went back into the office.

Making her way back outside, Eunny's grin widened. A confused sort of amusement built until she laughed outright. At herself, at Ollas's response. It felt like progress, and she felt more than satisfied. *Pleased.*

She shook her head at her silliness. They were well on their way to rekindling the friendship, that was all. It would make being back at Sylveren a lot more enjoyable, that was for sure, but the little flurry she was feeling about Ollas? Nothing.

Happiness at being real friends again. Just like it had been before. Good times. Which was all she wanted.

Her glow of delight flickered as she exited the tree. Almost against her will, she looked toward the greenhouse complex spread out around the Grove. Her gaze lingered on the furthest building. At this distance, the overgrown patch with its grassy clumps was barely visible, but her mind filled in the details.

"All right. First order of business then, buy gloves," she muttered. Thick ones, the kind that could grab a kettle off the stove without feeling a thing, because gods all break, she was keeping this job.

As she set off on the path back to town, the beginnings of a twitch tugged at the corner of her eye.

Chapter Six

Ignoring the pain in his leg, and his arm, and his side—his whole body, really—Ollas climbed the last few steps to the Grove's residential branch. He paused at the end of the hallway to catch his breath, gingerly kneading at his quaking thigh. Perhaps stealing down to the greenhouse complex hadn't been a great idea. He shrugged off his bag, grimacing as the motion pulled at his injured shoulder. He kept his fingers twined around the long strap so he wouldn't have to bend to retrieve it later. Chances were he'd end up collapsing on the floor and the sound would draw attention. If Eunny was around then she'd investigate, find out he'd been trying not to, as she put it, "let me earn my keep, Nev."

Which he was guilty of. But it had seemed silly to ask her to accompany him when he'd meant to just look over the materials Rai had brought in for the second trial. It wasn't meant to be a greenhouse tour. Ollas hadn't *meant* to linger. Eyes only. He hadn't unpacked the crates or anything! But Zhenya had come in while he was poking around, and *she'd* had some notes on potential first exercises for the elective, and his ten-minute trip had turned into almost two hours.

He'd never realized how uncomfortable the stools in the greenhouse were. The stabbing pain in his leg and side ensured he wouldn't soon forget.

Groaning, Ollas dragged himself the rest of the way to his door. He opened it as quietly as he could, peeking around the edge to scan the open living area. Empty. He sighed, tension draining away as he limped to his makeshift bed and eased himself down. He started to lift his bag up alongside, but the battered canvas, weighed down with soil samples and a book he wanted to review, ended up on the floor. He'd unpack it later. Maybe manage a quick nap before getting ready for the elective's first meeting that afternoon.

His eyes fluttered closed... and snapped open as the scrape of a key in the lock reached him.

Shit. Whichever of his roommates was on the other side, neither would be happy with his morning excursions. Despite his griping, Gransen treated Ollas like he was made of glass apt to shatter at the slightest provocation. And Eunny... Ollas didn't know what to do when it came to her. He probably should've asked her to accompany him earlier, but asking for help, for *her* help—the problem was twofold. His pride didn't want her to see him as something pitiable, and how could she not when she was waiting on him hand and foot? He was a walking reminder of yet another disaster that had befallen them.

A history that his cock didn't have nearly so many qualms about as his brain did, because it was still so delighted in her nearness that it threatened to embarrass him at any given moment.

And to what end? She'd said she wanted to help because she felt bad; a friend's guiltiness, nothing more. The night she'd shown up at his apartment, that momentary surprise when she'd seen him undressed, it had been just that—surprise. He was foolishly hopeful to think her easygoing nature could be anything else.

The door opened, and Eunny walked in.

"Hi," she said, already starting toward the connecting door to her quarters. She paused halfway there, taking in Ollas's disheveled appearance. "Where have you been?"

Ollas tried to haul himself more upright. "Nowhere. Just out for a—"

"You were out doing gardeny, *greenhousey* things, weren't you?" She pointed a mockingly accusatory finger at him, advancing a step with each word. "Without me."

"No," he protested, the word drawn out and weak and wholly unconvincing even to his own ears.

His good arm, weary from its morning activity and fatigued from having to do double duty, gave out. He lurched to the side, banging his injured limb against the shelving unit next to his bed. The wound pulled, a line of fire arcing along the barely healed flesh.

Ollas hissed in pain as he righted himself, clapping a hand over the sting pulsing outward from his arm. A trickle of wetness spread beneath his fingers. Probably not-so-healed, then. Great. Earthen fucking break him.

Eunny started forward, his name coming out as a startled cry.

He tried to wave her away. "I'm fine. I'm fine, really."

"Yea, the blood really sells it." She knelt beside the shelving unit and plucked up the bottle of healing salve the menders had sent him home with. She cast about for clean lint. "Please don't tell me you've been re-using that." She glowered at his bandage and its medley of colorful stains.

"Didn't want to waste the clean spots." Ollas tried to take the salve from her. "Eunny, you don't—"

"The Healing Hut has tons of the stuff," she said, referring to the House of Syvrine's healing ward by its more casual moniker. She unearthed a fresh roll of clean fabric and brandished it at him. "You look like shit. What were you doing earlier, trying to run?"

Ollas shrank back, shielding his arm from her. "Eunny, don't— It's…I can do it myself."

She rolled her eyes, hands lowering, but she didn't move away. "It's manual work, Ollas. I won't try to use my evil, dirty magic that I don't even have anymore on you."

"That's not—"

"Listen, I'm not actually saying this, but the gremlin isn't wrong in calling me your valet. Did we or did we not agree to that kind of arrangement?"

"Yes, but—"

Eunny tsked at him. "See, *yes*, we did. So, sneaking off instead of asking for help?" She thumped his bag. "Do I need to whack you on the nose with a scroll or something?"

Ollas's mouth opened, but no response came out. He didn't even know how to begin, to protest or apologize.

She raised the salve and lint again. "I know it's kind of weird being sort-of roommates. You don't have to like me being here, Ollas, but if I'm—"

"I do like you." The words slipped out, quiet and sure. Without any thought or worry at all. That part came after, as Eunny's eyes widened, her mouth frozen open.

Heat burned across Ollas's face, spurring him to babble on, "Living here. I like you living here. Being roommates, or whatever. I-I really appreciate it. You're—" In a detached way, a warning bell sounded in Ollas's head, trying to steer him to safer paths, but his mouth galloped on before his better sense caught up. "You're a good friend, Eunny."

Eunny's mouth slowly closed, her expression unreadable.

Ollas held back a despairing moan. His stupid mouth. Why did he have to say that...

"Oh?" she said, leaning toward him. In a conspiratorial whisper, she added, "Better than Gransen?"

A hoarse laugh bubbled out of him, and he gave her a weak smile. "You didn't hear it from me."

Eunny snorted, shaking her head as her eyes danced with glee. "Excuse you, but I'd like that in writing. I'm going to frame it and put it up over my door. No, his door. Humility would do him some good."

She reached slowly for his arm, eyebrows raised in question. Ollas nodded, grimacing as he held still.

Neither spoke as Eunny peeled away the dirty bandage, though she did hiss in sympathy as she cleansed the wound. It stung, but Ollas hardly noticed. It was taking every shred of his self-control not to do something pathetic like lean into her touch and blow the relaxed air between them all to hell.

Eunny re-wrapped his arm. "How does that feel? Better?"

"Much, thanks." Ollas cautiously rotated his arm. Still sore, but the fresh dressing helped.

"I can brew some tea that'll help with the tightness." Eunny stood up, gathering the pile of used bandages. "No magic, all from pre-made stores." She stuck her tongue out at him.

"Thanks," he repeated. As she turned away, he murmured, "Do you, back when—"

The door opened again, admitting Gransen. He glanced between the two of them. "Why, hello. Am I interrupting?"

"You should probably clean up," Eunny said. "You kind of smell like dirt, no offense, and I don't do bath duty."

Ollas blushed. "Yea, that's, I'll... Granse?"

Gransen saluted Eunny. "I'll scrub him raw in *all*—"

"I don't need the details." She glanced back at Ollas. "Were you going to ask something?"

"No, just..." Whatever brief bout of courage had risen in him, the moment for it had fled. "Thanks."

The corner of her mouth curled up. "I'll be back to help you with your stuff for class later."

~

I do like you.

Huh. Of course, he'd followed it up with the clarification of "living with her," and then capped it off with the death knell of being a "good friend." Which should've left Eunny feeling elated. Those words were incontrovertible proof of progress. And yet, she felt distinctly unsatisfied with them—those words, specifically—and couldn't quite put her finger on why.

Disgruntled, she sat back in her chair to watch the rest of the elective students trickle into the classroom. Zhenya had already been seated by the time Eunny and Ollas arrived. She'd claimed two small desks at the back of the room, and Eunny was grateful for the distance from the front, meager though it was. Sylveren had few large lecture halls, most of the class sizes being no larger than fifty. Twenty was the norm, and their current room in the Grove's classroom branch was sized to hold about that number.

Ollas had been quiet on their walk over, mumbling to himself every once in a while as he went over his introductory remarks. He probably could've managed just fine without her, but carrying his bag had given her an excuse to jest with him. He'd never be as brash as someone like Gransen, thank the gods. But he'd taken her teasing with good humor. Yes, he'd gone a bit blushy, but he also seemed relieved. More at ease around her than Eunny could remember him ever being in the last six years. A touch closer to who he'd been before the delegation's doomed rescue.

Professor Rai introduced himself, speaking for several minutes about the course and the syllabus. Eunny listened with half an ear as she watched the assembled students. Ollas had mentioned a mix of Initiate and Adept levels, and that was reflected in the fifteen people sitting in front of her. Mostly Initiate Fours and a handful of Adept Ones, if Eunny's judgment of age could be trusted. A mousy kid sat in the front row, watching the professors with rapt attention.

Ollas stood and traded places with Rai, his limp more pronounced as he walked the few steps without his cane.

He glanced at Eunny as he leaned against the room's large chalkboard before he looked out over the students. "As you can see, I had a little too much excitement before the start of term." His head dipped in a contrite nod, first toward Eunny and then at his bandages. "Miss Song will be helping out in the greenhouse as I recover."

Eunny gave the room a measured nod when Ollas motioned toward her.

"Went and broke your leg so you wouldn't have to haul dirt, Professor?" a redheaded young man joked.

Ollas stuck his hands in his pockets, an easy smile on his face. "Dirt?"

A few groans filled the air.

"You should know better by now, Lark," Ollas said. "Dirt. Does that really fit? I'm not trying to be pedantic." He waved down the scoffs that answered. "Dirt. That's a throwaway word. Simplistic. Calling it just 'dirt' doesn't really do justice to all that potential. The life. We're working with *soil*."

Beside her, Eunny could barely hear Zhenya murmur the word in tandem. Eunny bit down on her lip to stifle a laugh—or maybe it was a groan—good-natured though it was. Bless their plant-loving hearts.

"Soil is the foundation of this class. The seeds you'll work with, the plants and flowers we're hoping you can grow? The properties in them start in the ground first.

"Saren and I approved each and every one of you for acceptance into this elective. We know what you're capable of. You're here because you've been good. You're smart. You've all shown an aptitude for the material and sincerity for the cause. You wouldn't be here otherwise."

Ollas smiled, but solemnity kept it from brightening his eyes. "We're asking you to be better. You know what we're up against. We need your best, and for it to be more than what you've shown us before. It's a big ask. And it starts with the soil." This time, there was humor in his smile. "Because there's so much life in soil when it's treated right. It's easy—too easy—to strip the land down until it's just dirt. You've all taken the regenerative gardening prereq, you know that it takes work to maintain *soil*. Now, if you have seeds that want elevated heat and humidity to germinate, where should we start in building our starting mixes? Ennis?"

The mousy kid up front, Ennis, lowered their hand as they rattled off an argument for a named fire enchant Eunny had never heard of.

"Ollas loves this," Zhenya murmured, leaning forward to listen.

Eunny made a noise of agreement. She was fucking stunned. Where had *this* Ollas been the majority of the time she'd known him? She didn't know a damned thing about earth magic, yet he'd drawn her in. Had "dirt" halfway erased from her vocabulary.

Eunny found herself hanging on every word. Her mind raced with the possibilities for the elective's seeds, how she would devise a small test to grow her own. He had her thinking about what a starting mix should look like.

Ollas was in his element teaching, confident but easygoing,

encouraging the students to throw out suggestions. Even when they were off base, the way he corrected was kind. Informative while redirecting, never disdainful. Eunny watched him field questions, and something about his poise... it was magnetic.

Occasionally, he would meet her eye across the room, and—Was it her imagination or did his smile seem just a bit wider when that happened? That sensation of warmth fluttered across her skin, that *pleased* feeling she'd been experiencing around him. With him. From him? Pleased, and not in a platonic, celebration-of-a-friendship-saved kind of way. A *good friend,* as he'd called her. Which had been her goal, right? Signing herself up to help out for the elective, living in the room down the hall, all to help a friend.

But sitting there, catching those little smiles, their previous conversation rolling around in her head, Eunny felt that sense of dissatisfaction coming up again. Understood the emotion better now. Could do more than touch it with a finger. This side of Ollas—the calm, competent professor, building excitement and a belief in the magic of *soil* with his words—Eunny wanted more of it. To roll around in this feeling and clutch it to her chest and—

You broke him.

She balled her hands into fists.

No. Eunny couldn't let anything develop with Ollas. Foolish of her, getting carried away by a pretty speech. He had her thinking of magic. Of learning and possibility. Of a togetherness that Sylveren cultivated so well. A sense of optimism that he inspired with sheer enthusiasm. Gods, he'd almost caught her up in it, too.

Such feelings weren't for her. No community, no belonging. Eunny would do her part. Help Ollas with the manual labor. Do what she could to aid the secret priority of the elective, working on a cultivar that could help Dae's cause. Eunny owed them that. If she could help Dae up in Rhell, she would stick it out here to the bitter end.

But she would not let this become a place for her. She wouldn't delude herself that magic could be safe. Not ever again.

And Ollas, with his simple honesty—Eunny would watch herself with him, too. It was on her to atone, not for him to forgive. He was too nice, would forgive her gladly, and she deserved that least of all. She would have to endeavor not to forget it.

Chapter Seven

"You're welcome, by the way." Gransen raised his teacup in mock salute before taking a sip, aiming a pointed look at Ollas.

"For?" Ollas asked, already regretting taking the bait.

They'd survived the first week of fall term and had gone down to the Mighty Leaf to relax. Although Ollas's stubborn insistence on making use of one of the university's stable mounts had probably been foolhardy. Even kept to a walk, the motion of riding had aggravated the tweaked muscles in his back.

"Setting the stage so you can finally make your move. But oof, Olly. *Olly.* I didn't realize your path to love was going to be such an uphill battle."

"Shut up, Granse." Ollas cast a quick glance around their corner of the Mighty Leaf. Business was steady, many of the tables filled by an even split of Sylvan locals and university folk in need of new surroundings for their weekend studies. The buzz of a dozen conversations filled the air, Ollas and Gransen's no more remarkable than any other. "It's not uphill."

"Did Eunny kiss your boo-boo to make it all better? Ruffle your hair and chuck you under the chin?"

Ollas made a rude gesture at him.

Gransen laughed. "So, how's it going, pining after my boss?"

Wonderful. Horrible. "She's not your—"

"It's an informal agreement. Stop stalling, Nevin."

Nevin, but not Nev. Which was good; Ollas didn't want Eunny's shorthand being appropriated by anyone else.

He bounced between the euphoria of having Eunny around all the time, suffused in her exuberance and sharp wit, and the despair of knowing Eunny's jokes were just Eunny being herself. A manifestation of her outgoing nature, harmless, good fun. Friendliness, but not flirtation. Not with Ollas.

How long had he nursed his unrequited love? He'd been intrigued, awed, by her as a kid. But true attraction, that had grown a little slower. He'd admired her fierce loyalty. To a shy town boy, seeing a tween outsider, a slip of a girl, get into shouting matches with grown men who dared to hassle her aunt and disparage the Mighty Leaf had blown young Ollas away. But they'd only been kids. A boy's infatuation. What of the man?

"It's— It's not, I guess. I didn't know we were even friends until Initiate Two," Ollas murmured.

"That's okay. Leave it to Papa Gransen to—"

"Not a word." Ollas pointed at him. "Not one—"

Gransen gave a short, low whistle, his gaze focused on a point behind Ollas's head. "Look alive, Olly." He waved, calling out, "Hey, boss!"

Eunny made a face at him as she came over. "We've talked about that. You'd have to work for me—"

"I willingly subject myself to your abuse on a weekly basis."

"You don't get paid. You're not an employee."

"Oh, Eun, we don't deal in anything so crass as *money*."

Gransen dismissed her words with a shrug. "Speaking of, when can I get back in there?"

Eunny rubbed her temples. "I've barely had a chance to go through the salvage piles."

"Let me. I'm the manager, let me *manage.*" Gransen made a flourish with his hands.

Their argument over duties to Song's Scrap—real or otherwise—were called to a halt when Eunny's aunt Yerina came over.

"Hello, Ollas, dear," she murmured as she hugged him, mindful of his tender arm. "For your mama." She pressed a small bag of tea into his hand.

Straightening, Yerina looked to her niece. The older woman was usually so warm and cheery, but now, concern dimmed her eyes, and a frown line marred her round face. "Eunny, the new distributor from Central District I've been in talks with came up early."

"That's fine. I can hang around until you're done, or I can come back later to—" Eunny squinted at her aunt's wary expression. "What's wrong?"

"I didn't know that a representative from the Coalition would be coming up with them," Yerina said.

"Didn't you just have your check-in with them last..." Eunny's eyes widened. Then narrowed, her expression going flat. "You mean *she's* here."

Yerina nodded. "Stay, please? It's been so long." She gave her niece an imploring look.

Gransen raised his hand. "Who's *she?*"

"Ah, there they are. Yerina, what are you— Oh. This is a surprise." A short exhale, somewhere between a sigh and a false laugh, sounded behind them. "Gentlemen, I don't believe you've met my daughter, Eunji."

Even if she'd never spoken, Ollas couldn't mistake the

woman striding toward them as anyone other than Eunny's mother. Same athletic build and same oval face with soft features, though Eunny's chin leaned toward stubborn. Where Eunny's dark hair skimmed her shoulders, her mother's was long, its gentle waves reaching her ribs.

Everything about the woman marked her as someone from Graelynd's Central District. Her black cloak bore a glimmer of silk blended with fine wool. She wore a long black dress as well, the draping fabric tailored to fit. Her only accessory was a silver belt woven from wires scarcely larger than thread.

A glamorous figure, and cold. As she made the flurry of introductions, Ollas tried to reconcile the image of the woman before him with the one from a memory now six years old. Bioon Song hadn't been so coiffed the only other time they'd met. No, she'd been bruised and worn, as so many of the delegation had been by the time Ollas's Sentinels group rescued them. But her eyes. The way she always seemed to be analyzing everything, *everyone,* measuring their value. That hadn't changed. It created such a stark contrast between her and both her daughter and sister. Yerina's face bore laugh lines, her hair touched with gray, but even when she was tired from a busy day at the tearoom, she always possessed an aura of joy. Bioon Song seemed like the kind of person whose smile never touched her eyes.

Yerina hesitated at the table's edge, murmuring to Eunny that it wouldn't take long. Bioon shooed her sister away. "There's no rush. I have business matters to discuss while I'm here." She waited until her colleagues and sister had departed before turning her full attention to Ollas and his friends.

"Ollas Nevin, the Homegrown Hero. It's been a while."

"Ma'am." He glanced sidelong at Eunny, who was regarding her mother with thinly veiled suspicion. "You seem well."

"I'm glad you're here. Thought I'd have to trek up to the

university to find you." Bioon offered a polite smile to Gransen, but her mouth twitched with something like scorn as she regarded her daughter. "I represent an interest in one of Ollas's classes this fall. Would you mind if we spoke privately?"

Gransen shifted in his chair. Eunny dug around in her bag and produced a key. She handed it to him. "Go manage."

Gransen took the key to the repair café and beat a hasty retreat. Ollas watched him go, a sinking feeling in his stomach as mother and daughter stared at one another.

"What are you doing here?" Eunny asked, voice low but blunt.

Bioon tutted. "Is that any way to greet your mother?"

Eunny didn't answer, merely raised her eyebrows in perfect imitation of the expectant look Bioon gave her.

"My business is with Ollas," Bioon said. She leaned toward him, murmuring, "I thought I'd done her a favor, not insisting on the same strict filial piety norms of other Hanyeok parents. Perhaps I was mistaken."

"So you've said before," Eunny muttered. "You're one to talk. When was the last time you saw either of *your* parents?"

"You mentioned something about the school?" Ollas cut in. "Eunny is helping me with my workload for a bit." He indicated his injured limbs.

"My sympathies. I hope you recover quickly." Bioon settled back in her chair, signaling to a passing server to bring more tea. "Very well. Eunji, this meeting isn't to be fodder for any town gossip."

Eunny gave her mother a sour smile. "Because I make a habit of mongering rumors."

Ignoring her daughter, Bioon pointedly faced Ollas. "I'm facilitating for the Restorers of the Alliance and their business ventures as they pertain to Coalition interests."

"Okay," Ollas said, feeling lost.

"What does that have to do with Sylveren?" Eunny asked.

"The elective Ollas is teaching with Professor Rai. The Coalition is coming on board as a sponsor." Bioon pulled an unsealed letter from her cloak pocket and placed it on the table.

Ollas skimmed the letter, while Eunny leaned closer to read over his shoulder. It contained the usual directives for regular reporting, a summarized calendar of disbursements from the Coalition, and shipping schedules. It didn't seem all that different from other outside funding arrangements that took place at the school, aside from an excess of verbiage for nondisclosure. The delivery timetable was ridiculous, wanting weekly samples sent to the Coalition headquarters down in Graelynd; even with arcane enhancements to speed plant growth, it was unrealistic to think they'd have anything worth showing for weeks. Still, it wasn't a major inconvenience if the Coalition was willing to pay the shipping fees, and the seals on the documentation were legitimate.

A server brought a fresh pot of tea while Ollas read. Eunny returned to the cup she'd poured for herself upon arriving, though she seemed to fiddle with it more than drink as she watched her mother. Bioon sipped her tea, the picture of calm.

"Everything in order?" she asked at last. "I can bring any questions you have back to Central."

"No, ma'am, this is easy enough," Ollas murmured, "but the request for weekly samples, it's, ah, excessive. In the early stages, we won't have anything worth sending."

"Why is the Coalition being so micromanaging?" Eunny said.

"Standard procedure in all Coalition business." Bioon's eyes flicked toward her daughter. "Of course, seeing as this is our first partnership with Sylveren, perhaps we'll need to adjust. The Coalition has high hopes for this enterprise's success. I'll suggest to my colleagues that we establish more frequent in-person meetings in lieu of the weekly samples. I'll personally see to it. Does that sound agreeable?"

Ollas couldn't tell if Bioon expected a response from him, given the way she was smiling at her daughter. Not a smirk, nothing so obvious as that, but a perfectly shaped curl to her mouth that was visually acceptable yet screamed of insincerity.

Eunny had no reservations about hiding her suspicion. She crossed her arms over her chest. "You hate the Valley and it hates you. Why would you volunteer to come here more often?"

"I have family here, Eunji. Wouldn't it be nice to see each other more often?"

"You've never tried before," Eunny muttered.

Bioon continued as if Eunny hadn't spoken. "I admit, I'm surprised to see you attaching yourself to this project," she said. "Considering that it—"

"I live here. I have business with the school from time to time." Eunny gave an indifferent shrug.

"Business hasn't been going so well here, though, has it?"

Eunny flushed.

"I saw your little... *shop.*" A tiny smile traced Bioon's lips before her expression returned to neutral. "Unfortunate. It's quite lucky, really, that you could attach yourself to the elective."

"I asked," Ollas said, cutting Eunny off from what threatened to be a shouted reply. "I could use her help."

"Help from someone with no grovetending expertise? Why, she's not even interested in gardening, unless"—Bioon glanced at Eunny—"your hobbies have dramatically changed?"

"The course benefits from other perspectives," Ollas said. "And it's only a few weeks while I—"

"It isn't difficult for you, daughter, given the subject matter?" Bioon's eyes never left Eunny. "A curative for the new complications up north. It would be a shame if your emotions affected the coursework."

"I'm so touched by your concern," Eunny said sourly, resting her elbows on the table. "Is that why you're here? The Coalition wants in on any curatives we produce? You here to make sure the Coalition gets its cut? Gods all break if we actually help people without maximizing Coalition profits."

"*We* produce?" Bioon's head tilted as though she were a bird studying potential prey. "I thought you were only temporary help. Are you finally working on recovering your magic? How responsible of you."

"That's not what I said."

"It's about time. Six years of hiding." Bioon shook her head, eyes going to Ollas once more. "It's my fault. I should've insisted on more therapy and immersion from the start. Letting her fear just fester like this—"

"I'm not afraid!" Eunny snapped, earning a few surprised looks from other patrons. She ducked her head, continuing in a furious whisper, "I *lost* my magic. It's gone, Mother. No amount of wishful thinking on your part will change that."

"You don't just lose magic, Eunji. It's not the key to your house. It's repressed within you, only you're too scared—"

"When did you become a scholar of traumatic incidents? You don't know what you're talking about. You don't even have magic."

Ollas had never seen Eunny like this. She griped about Gransen on occasion, even snapped at him when he was being particularly single-minded about something she didn't want for the café. But this jagged, emotional reaction, the quick, defensive anger? The only other time he could recall anything similar was at the Mighty Leaf's solstice release earlier that summer. Tourists harping on at Eunny about the kidnapping, the rescue, how lucky she was that the Homegrown Hero was still friendly with the Healer Who Hurts.

It wasn't a memory he enjoyed. He'd never given it any further thought, the way Eunny was so adamant about her lack of fear when it came to magic. She was so quick to refute, and maybe that hinted at something deeper than the bad faith between mother and daughter. Although, witnessing the bitter dynamic between them, Ollas could hardly blame Eunny for her reticence.

Bioon unnerved him, no question, but Eunny's distress did something to his insides. Had that protective flame burning hot.

"Since my own grasp of magic is pretty weak, we're a good pair," Ollas said, overriding Bioon's reply. "Eunny's knowledge of body magic is really helpful in devising soil mixes and evaluation results. I'm optimistic about the trials we have planned."

Bioon regarded him with a cool glance, expression giving nothing away.

Nervous sweat broke out across his palms at the older woman's scrutiny. He tried to nonchalantly wipe them on his trousers, making a show of repositioning his bad leg. "Sylveren prides itself on providing our students with both magic-born and mundane perspectives, so they have a well-rounded education."

"Well said." Bioon's lips morphed into a smile, her tone back to light, almost playful. "He's good for you, Eunji."

"He's a good friend," Eunny replied, the words sounding almost like a challenge. "Always has been."

It was a compliment, yet it made Ollas want to shrivel up inside. A good friend. His own words come back to mock him. That was Ollas, her childhood pal. Could nicer, more unromantic words be used to describe him?

Bioon looked over Ollas's shoulder. "My employers have

high hopes for the elective. Come say hello to my colleagues here. I'm sure they'd love any insights you can share, a little something to take back to their superiors in Central, hmm?"

Ollas fixed his polite, Homegrown-Hero-appeasing-the-masses smile on his face. Years of teaching, not to mention the hours he'd spent practicing and refining the look in the mirror, let it come naturally. Handy to have it in his back pocket.

He chanced a sidelong glance at Eunny. The minute motion of her jaw suggested she was chewing a hole in her lip to keep from speaking.

Ollas feigned a grimace. Let his injured shoulder quiver as he lifted his hands in an apologetic gesture. "I'm so sorry, Ms. Song, but I've about reached my excitement level for the day."

"You poor dear," Bioon said. "That must be difficult."

"Yea, speaking of, we should grab a carriage for the trip," Eunny said. "We have class prep to do still. Need you conscious for it."

"Good idea."

Bioon stood. "I'll take my leave as well." She consulted a gold pocket watch. "We may be able to take the next windrunner back."

"You're not going to see Aunt Yerina?" Eunny asked, appalled.

Bioon gave her an unreadable look, then turned toward her colleagues as they waited at the front of the tearoom. "We saw each other."

The Graelynders left first, Bioon sparing only a few words for her sister before she walked out. Yerina watched her go, sorrow on her face. She patted Eunny's cheek in farewell before disappearing into the Mighty Leaf's back room.

"Do you want to stay?" Ollas asked. "I'll be fine on my own."

Eunny shook her head. "No, we'll just argue. I'll come down

later to make it up to her." She gave him a wry smile. "Thanks though. I appreciate the thought."

That was him, *a good friend,* through and through. A good friend, but hardly a close one. As Ollas followed Eunny outside, he wondered what he could do to remove that gap. To become more than platonic in her eyes. Only, his babbling mouth had already put the *good friend* notion in her head, and he didn't know how to get it out.

Chapter Eight

THE RIDE back to the university passed quietly, Ollas sitting across from Eunny in the small carriage as she stared out the window. Ollas looked down at his lap, at his hands curled into useless fists. He was desperate to break the silence, but unsure of what to say. How to address the discomfort of what had happened? Or was it better to pretend, ignore?

"Your mother seems..." He paused, fumbling for a word.

Eunny faced him, a wry smile tugging at her lips.

"Cold," he said.

She let out a bark of laughter. "As a fish. She's a coldhearted bitch, Nev, and she's the first to admit it."

"Did she even answer any of your questions about the Coalition?"

"She doesn't answer anything she doesn't want to. She's an expert at that," Eunny muttered.

"I'm sorry things are so...I don't know. I'm just sorry, I guess."

"Don't be. Besides, damn, Nev! You *lied*." Eunny leaned across the carriage to poke him in his good shoulder. "I didn't think you had it in you."

He ducked his head to hide his grin. "Hard to believe she and Yerina are sisters."

"I feel bad for my aunt. I walked away a long time ago, but she still tries to have us be her idea of a family." Eunny sobered, weariness stealing across her face. "The Mighty Leaf was supposed to be a joint venture or something, but Bioon didn't care. She hates the Valley, and a teashop didn't exactly fit her power-hungry lifestyle. But I can't convince my auntie that Bioon is a lost cause."

Ollas shook his head. His ma didn't see her older brother much now that he'd moved down to Graelynd, but they corresponded with regularity. The coldness Eunny spoke of—and to someone as welcoming as Yerina—baffled him.

"I don't trust her," Eunny said quietly. "My mother. I don't know enough about the Restorers to judge, but I'm suspicious of the Coalition just on principle. If my mother's here repping them, and especially with how quick she was to volunteer to come up, *to the Valley,* in person? They're up to something."

"The school won't let them meddle. They won't," Ollas insisted at her dubious look. "The school doesn't bow to Grae-lynd's whims, and I don't think even the Coalition will want to fight with the Order. And they *will* get involved if anyone tries to exert influence that's against the school's values."

The Order of Sylveren, the ruling council for the entire valley, ensured that the region's stance as a neutral zone—open to all regardless of nationality, provided they came with good-will—was respected. Rarely did they need to enforce such matters with violence, but the region's history was marked with such events. When the Order acted, they did so swiftly, thoroughly, and even countries further abroad than Graelynd remembered. Not even the warlords of Eylle had tried to take on the Valley after their first attempt centuries ago was slapped down. If a kingdom as volatile as Eylle didn't dare to mess with the Valley, Ollas didn't think Graelynd's governing body of trade would, either.

Eunny hummed in consideration. "That'd be something." She shrugged, her expression still grim. "Wouldn't put it past them to still try, though, at least until they get caught. The Coalition cares about money more than anything else. A cure for the poison could be worth a lot."

"Rhell's not rolling in gold after the war and six years of their land being wrecked by the corruption."

"Maybe I should've said value. Rhell has a wellspring, Graelynd doesn't. I mean, it does fine with the way the ley lines run, since it gets to be the Valley Junior, but the Coalition is always looking for more. More, I don't know… Just, *more*." Eunny was looking out the window again, but she seemed lost in memory. "That's what the delegation was, I'm almost certain of it."

"What do you mean?"

She shook her head, gaze still unfocused, looking deep into her past. "A *trade* delegation, between Eylle and the Coalition? They don't care about each other or mending fences. That's politicking for the Councils. I mean, I believe that the Coalition wanted assurances in place for smooth trading, but I always figured that the Coalition was really just looking to get Graelynd officially into the war."

Ollas nodded along; it made sense, seeing as Graelynd boasted an impressive navy. Once deployed, Eylle couldn't match it, especially so far from the empire's waters.

Eunny shrugged. "But when I was there, before they kidnapped us in place and didn't let anyone leave, it felt like the Eyllics *were* there to deal, but something changed."

"A different deal than trade?"

"Maybe. Or different trading than I was led to believe, but then again, Mother Dearest didn't actually inform me of much. I expected there to be a lot more paper-shuffling, though. They wanted…" Eunny broke off, hiding a grimace with a shake of her head. "I can't really remember. Those were shit times. All I'll say is that the Coalition doesn't care about *good* or *right for the world*, just for themselves. If others benefit, that's nice and all, but they're looking out for themselves first."

Ollas didn't know what to say. It was the most he'd ever heard Eunny say of her time with the delegation. It felt like a chance to do some explaining of his own, despite the bitter sort of finality with which she'd spoken—the window of opportunity, if he was going to take it, already beginning to close. They were in a carriage, no interruptions present. The school was still a few minutes away. Nothing but silence and dwindling opportunities between them. Hadn't he come back to Sylveren to try and make amends, start something new?

"I'm sorry," he murmured. "About what happened to the delegation. I'm sorry for my part in it."

Eunny swung around to face him, confusion on her face. "What are you talking about?"

"It's my fault." Ollas looked down at his hands clasped atop his knee. He steeled himself, forced a steadying breath. This had gone on far too long. "I found signs in the woods, thought it was poachers. I'm the one who insisted to my group that we follow them. We found this cache, and I was digging through it when the fight started. I broke protocol—I just ran out there after the noise. If I hadn't done that, if I hadn't gotten hurt, or at least stopped you from—"

"Hold on." Eunny raised a hand to stop him. "You're apologizing because your actions led to me and a bunch of others being *rescued? From Eyllic kidnappers?*" Her voice rose with each word.

"I— Yes?" Ollas said, wary. "That's kind of simplifying it a—"

"If you hadn't, we'd still be *kidnapped,* you dolt." Her hands shook as she gestured emphatically, nearly hitting him in the close quarters of the carriage.

"Yes, well, no, but I mean, it's my fault because I didn't stop you! I-I screwed up your magic," Ollas protested. "I knew you were tired, but when you tried to heal me, I just... And then your magic—"

"Ollas, you didn't make that happen. It— It got away from me. That's not your fault." Eunny reached out and pressed her hand against his mouth when he tried to speak. "Listen to me. It's. Not. Your. Fault. No one blames you, least of all me."

"You should," he whispered, and steeled himself to admit the rest. How he'd wanted to feel her magic, to know that side of Eunny Song. His once-in-a-lifetime chance, or so he'd thought. "Do you re—"

She pressed her finger against his lips. "If anything, you should hate *me*. I'm the Healer Who Hurts, remember?" Though her tone was light, the smile she gave him was sad.

"Never," Ollas said. "I've never hated you. Never blamed you, either. I just... I don't know what to say. Whenever that day gets mentioned, you're pretty quick to shut it down. Understandably," he added.

Her lips twitched, more grimace than smile. "I can talk about it, in general. But no, I don't love being asked to recount how it felt to have my magic go rogue. I'm not lying when I say I don't remember much of that day. When I try, it's... unpleasant." Her gaze went unfocused again, as if she was looking into the past and not at the carriage wall. "Doesn't put me in a rush to try and get it back. It was the worst day of my life, Nev, but none of that's on you."

"Even though—"

She took one of his hands between hers, leaning closer to meet his eyes. "I *am* grateful that you still want to be friends.

More than you can ever know. I don't know that I deserve it, but can we just go on from that?"

Ollas wanted to refute her points, convince her that she deserved everything. Happiness. Peace. Desperation and despair spiraled through him at her gentle, *relieved* affirmation of friendship. All he could muster was a soft, "Okay."

"Good." Eunny sat up, her manner morphing from solemn to light and brisk once more. "Glad that's settled."

"Do you ever miss it?" he asked, hesitant but curious. "Grae-lynd. Your life there?"

"Not really. Living in Central is..." Eunny wrinkled her nose in thought, then shrugged. "It takes a certain kind of personality. I made better friends during my summers up here anyway, Dae excluded, but she was so wrapped up in her old life there, too, that we didn't see each other much even when we lived in the same city. And the work—well, I couldn't have opened the café down there. Not the style."

The carriage rolled to a stop at the stable area below Sylveren University's main courtyard.

"You up for finally giving me the greenhouse tour?" she asked.

Eunny and her way of moving, practically *barreling* on. She shrugged off the heaviness of their conversation, not with flippancy but with a surety that left him standing in her wake. He was stunned, maybe a bit confused, definitely unnerved.

"Sure," Ollas said, somewhat dazed as he reached for the door lever located on the side of his bad arm.

"Here, Nev, let me help."

"It's okay, I can manage a door."

Only, the word "door" ended more as a yelp when it opened with less resistance than he'd expected. Ollas couldn't get a hand free, limbs tangling with his cane in the tight confines of the carriage. Oh, gods all break. He was going to fall on his face.

Tear something. Maybe break a bone while he was at it, and wouldn't that just—

Arms encircled his waist, caught him, and heaved him back, a muffled grunt sounding at his ear though the motion was smooth. Eunny's was a firm, solid kind of strength that denied gravity, that pulled him not simply into the carriage but farther, until they thumped onto the narrow bench.

Ollas was pressed against Eunny's chest. Was engulfed by her, as if her body endeavored to wrap around him: one hand was snug around his middle while the other reached past to brace against the carriage's side panel.

It should've alarmed him, being sprawled across Eunny like that. Being held. Ollas had hugged people before—hard not to, when his mother had all but made a sport out of it. He'd been intimately embraced before, too. If there was a perk to being dubbed the Homegrown Hero, it was that it had garnered him some interest, let him hone a few carnal skills. Yet none of those acquaintances had made his heartbeat speed like it did now, and not from nearly falling out of a carriage but because every fiber of his being was acutely aware that Eunny Song was holding him with such casual ease.

A jiggling motion at his back made Ollas freeze. Then the sound of her poorly concealed laughter nearly turned him to jelly.

"Can manage a door, eh?" Eunny let go, gently pushing him up. "You're squishing me."

"Sorry," Ollas said, heat burning across his cheeks as he stumbled onto the opposite bench. "Oh, gods, I'm so, so— Eunny, are you— I'm *so* sorry."

Eunny waved away his stammering apologies, her grin turning more into a smirk. "I'm hardly fragile. Calm down, Nev. Wasn't going to let you break again on my watch." She reached past him to push the door fully open. "Let me get the stool," she said, laughter in her voice.

Eunny wasn't upset. No, even better, she was joking with him. Felt enough at ease to make light of *that* part of their past. It was as if the final piece of ice between them had finally broken away, the tension and regret banished. Like they could truly pick up, now, from where their relationship had been. Not running from the past but no longer being held back by it, either.

Maybe his babble was finally setting him on a better course.

The thought filled him with relief. With hope. Made a tremor run down his spine. And... had his cock bobbing against the confines of his trousers, a mortifying realization as he tried to will it into submission, or at the very least compliance—as he tried to say something, anything, that would distract Eunny from noticing. All that came out was an incoherent squeak. When words failed, he went with what he knew. Used his cloak as a shield, pretending to fuss with his cane as he flipped his cock up beneath his waistband. Treacherous fucking thing.

Eunny didn't seem any the wiser as she helped him down, bowing over his hand with an exaggerated flourish.

They struck off down the path to the greenhouse complex, side by side.

Eunny liked to think she was in decent shape. Not up for running with the Sentinels anytime soon, but she trekked around town often enough. Helped out in the Mighty Leaf regularly, both with serving and the manual labor of unpacking shipments. Not to mention all the lifting, carrying, crouching. Gods all break, so much crouching and kneeling involved in her repair café work. The point was, Eunny was active.

Or so she thought. They'd been working in Trunk, the storage greenhouse, for a couple hours now, and Eunny's back and feet were starting to hurt. She was even beginning to get a blister on her palm from gripping the wheelbarrow handles too tight. A blister! As if she didn't use her damned hands every day for work already.

"You really don't need to bring any more in," Ollas said, an apologetic note in his voice.

He sat perched on a stool at a workbench that spanned the length of the greenhouse wall. Piles of different soil mixes and amendments covered the surface, while large wooden bins on wheels, each housing a different component, surrounded him. Several more of the bins were tucked beneath the bench, some empty and others already labeled and filled with special blends.

Eunny lugged two more bags over to the bench and added them to the stack she'd been growing. "All right. I'm now fully in favor of making the students haul their own dirt." She exhaled with much drama to emphasize her point.

"It's so—"

"Hush, you."

Snagging her own stool, she flopped down, leaning back so her elbows rested on the countertop. Her arms quaked with fatigue. They'd intended to just have a quick look around the greenhouse complex, but one question had led to a demonstration, which had then turned into Ollas going into prep mode. Nettled as she was about her body's weaknesses, Eunny was glad she'd asked for the orientation. The elective had magic-users and mundane alike, and a wide variety of imbued amendments available for them to try, courtesy of more funding from the Restorers and a sponsorship from Graelynd contacts.

Ollas had a lot of preparations he'd still wanted to do for the elective before their first lab, and he wasn't in any condition to be doing so much heavy lifting. Over the last couple of hours,

Eunny had become well-versed in some basic greenhouse jargon and learned more about the focus of each building in the complex than she'd ever need to know.

She watched as Ollas mixed the components from a few bags and bins he'd assembled while she'd been ferrying around the sacks of dirt. Along with the dirt she'd hauled in, he used measuring scoops to add powders and granules to a large tub, even chucking in what looked like sand and some handfuls of moss. Then he combined everything together, nodding toward a watering can as he looked at Eunny. "Could you pour while I mix?"

She grabbed the can and wetted down the medley of dirt as Ollas turned it over with a hand trowel and then a small rake.

"Is this for the class?" She pointed with her chin toward a new blend.

"It'll be their baseline." Ollas scooped it into an empty bin. "They'll make more throughout the course and start developing their own changes."

Eunny eyed a row of seed-starting trays he'd lined up against the wall. "Are you doing all of those now?"

"No, they can wait."

As Eunny helped him stow everything away, a group of Adept Two grovetenders and their Magister Three-level supervisor came in to gather supplies. With the door to the front antechamber propped open and a few of the big rolling bins of potting mix blocking off the main entrance, Ollas gestured toward the back of Trunk. Brushing aside a few dangling vines that had crawled through gaps between the antechamber walls and the greenhouse's roof, Eunny pushed open the heavy back door so they could make their escape.

"Sorry, this didn't end up being very quick," Ollas said.

"It was good. I did ask to be orientated." Eunny bumped his shoulder. "But I'm beat—"

A low pulling sensation wrapped around a corner of her mind. It set off a pulse at her temple, near her eye but not quite the same twitching she'd felt on previous occasions. It wasn't painful but... insistent. Impossible to ignore.

Looking around, Eunny swallowed down a curse. When they'd first arrived at Trunk, she had surreptitiously steered Ollas's tour so that they gave the overgrown patch along the side of the building a wide berth. The grassy clumps dotted a narrow plot at the back of the greenhouse, sweeping out from the door to curve around the corner. She'd assumed they were weeds, but in daylight Eunny noticed they were contained, somewhat, to a specific area. Intentionally planted, then, though not very well maintained. And she still didn't have gloves.

Carefully shutting the greenhouse door, she crossed her arms, keeping her hands well clear of the plants. "We should—"

Ollas wasn't listening. Head cocked toward the plants, he made an intrigued sound at the back of his throat. He stepped to the edge of the narrow path, using his cane for leverage so he could stiffly crouch down. Uncaring of the light rain falling, he lifted his arm, one hand outstretched toward the nearest damned plant.

"Nev, don't!" Eunny started forward, the feeling of being drawn next to him in conflict with an instinctive need to drag him away.

Ollas's head swiveled around, his hazel eyes widening with surprise. "You can feel it, too?"

Shit. Eunny pulled her hands back, stuffing them into her cloak's pockets instead of dragging Ollas away. Or worse— giving in to the irrational pull urging her to step into the grassy patch.

"I... No. Feel what?" she said in a rush.

Ollas had already turned back to survey the plants. "I found these as seeds during the rescue. In the camp." Wariness crossed his face as he glanced at her, then back at the plants. He reached out and ran his fingers along one of the long, strappy leaves. "It— It's like they're calling to us."

"That's ridiculous, Ollas," Eunny said with more force than she'd intended. "I'd need magic for that, and I don't have it anymore, remember?"

He shrugged, the harsh edge in her voice apparently going unnoticed. "Maybe they're imbued. I planted these years ago and they never... Maybe it's the conditions changing. I need to check..." He blinked, as if realizing he was muttering nonsense to himself. A sheepish grin spread across his face. "Sorry. Got carried away."

"Come on, plant boy. You're going to get your bandages wet." Eunny offered him her hand, mindful to keep herself safely on the path.

Ollas groaned softly as he righted himself, stretching out his knee. He staggered a step, and Eunny tightened her grip to steady him. "Thanks," he said, a hint of pink rising in his cheeks.

Eunny smiled up into his face, a breezy comment on the tip of her tongue. When had he gotten so tall? Enough that she had to raise her chin, anyway. Maybe he always had been, and they'd just never been so close. Close to the point where Eunny could see that he had a dusting of freckles across his nose and cheeks. Strange. They'd known each other for literal decades by now, had been in close proximity before, even if not often. Yet, she'd never noticed he possessed freckles.

In a vague sense, Eunny knew she was staring. But so was he, eyes wide and unblinking as they met hers. He blushed deeper this time, seemed in a quandary over whether to drop her hand or gently let go. He settled for handing it back to her, movements stilted but somehow endearing. It drew a sputter from her, a half-choked laugh that she tried and failed to hold back.

Ollas ducked his head, shoulders rounding toward his ears. He'd grown into those, too—the shoulders and the ears. The former had a nice bit of muscle now instead of being all youthful boniness. The ears, eh, they'd always kind of stuck out, and not even his dark curls could hide that. But on Adult Ollas, they lent a bit of charm.

Charm? Gods all break her. Eunny was certain she'd never once thought of Ollas Nevin as charming in her entire life. Yet, somehow, she was thinking charitable thoughts about him. And... if she was honest with herself, those kinds of thoughts had been increasing of late. Which wasn't such a bad thing, was it? He wasn't exactly running screaming in the other direction, so there surely wasn't any harm in testing the proverbial waters.

He's good for you, Eunji.

Her mother's approval was enough to snap Eunny back to her senses. She would *not* have those kinds of thoughts about Ollas. Flattering ones. The kind that viewed him in any other light than platonic. She liked him as a friend. Anything more was undeserved. More than she could ever ask. Bad enough to be the Healer Who Hurts—she couldn't be with the one she'd damaged. That wasn't why she was here.

How responsible of you, Bioon had said. A subtle dig at Eunny's supposed sense of duty and the selfishness that had taken its place. Eunny wasn't about to try and change it. Had spent the last six years ridding herself of those kinds of attachments, save for a precious few that she trusted to be safe. Auntie Yerina, Dae, Zhenya, maybe even Gransen, that little shit. People she could safely care about because they put no expectations on her aside from friendship. Those relationships had no hidden asks, no demands for more than Eunny could comfortably give.

Ollas straddled a line between friendship and something else. Something alluring, and all the more dangerous for it. So sweet and unassuming, he should've been easy for Eunny to banish. She'd never given Kid Ollas a second thought. But now? Ollas had grown, and she was liking the adult version more than she ought. An attraction that needed to be smushed. She wasn't sticking around here for long; their arrangement was only good until Ollas was fully back on his feet. Even healing at a normal, unassisted-by-magic rate, it wouldn't take more than a few weeks.

"We should probably, you know..." Eunny jerked her head in the direction of the Grove.

"Yea. I think I should give my leg a break, too," Ollas mumbled, shifting his grip on his cane.

As they left Trunk behind, Eunny chattered about nothing, wrangling the shameless part of her that wanted to luxuriate in the memory of Ollas pressed against her in the carriage, the appeal of his freckles, just...everything about him, really. She gathered the feeling up and threw it in a mental cage through sheer force of will.

Maybe her mother was right and Ollas could be good for Eunny, but she'd never let herself find out. She was just here to help him keep his job, and then she'd be gone. Back to her repair café. The life that she...liked, mostly. Had chosen for herself. She'd go back, as planned, and that was that.

Chapter Nine

Do you ever miss it? Graelynd. Your life there?

Eunny's life in Graelynd had revolved around her mother's Coalition work, even as she'd scratched and fought for every scrap of distance between them she could get. Hard to escape Bioon's long shadow, though, even when Eunny's apothecary practice seemingly had no connection to her. But the politicking of Central District was bad enough, and that would've been without having Bioon as a mother. The nature of Eunny's small-time apothecary work back then was always at odds with the lifestyle and interests of Central folk. She might have felt a few regretful, nostalgic pangs for the idea of it, working with herbs and finding the best ways to help an individual's little hurts, but the reality of her old life held nothing of note. And with regard to her life now, *right now,* Eunny hadn't seen it coming.

A week passed, one blurring into two and then three. The days took on a steady rhythm of mornings spent helping Ollas to his Initiate One class—Introduction to Arcane Agroecology, which Eunny usually sat in on—or the elective, depending on the day. Most afternoons went to greenhouse work. Since Ollas didn't need her for his office hours, Eunny usually lazed around the apartment and caught up on her reading. She'd meant to use the time to do some research on better repair techniques for when she had to return to Song's Scrap and the mountain of overdue work. What had survived the collapse, anyway.

Except it was hard to drum up enthusiasm for such an endeavor. Which was how she found herself asking more about the elective and the horticulture side of it. Ollas suggested an herbalism textbook, and what started out as idle curiosity grew into something more dedicated while Ollas was away at his office hours. It was just to make her more efficient while she helped out, Eunny told herself. Nothing professional, nothing like apothecary work. Strictly gardening know-how. This interest she felt in reading a *textbook* of all things, it was just... nostalgia. Apothecary work was something she'd thought would be her life. Completely normal to feel a feeling when revisiting it.

The apartment door opened, pulling Eunny from her jumble of thoughts as Gransen arrived home from class.

"Coming back to the dark side?" he said, sliding into a seat across from her at the kitchen table.

Eunny shut the book. "Gremlin. No, just something Nev recommended."

"Nev." Gransen rested his chin in his hands, elbows propped on the table as he grinned at her. "So cute how you have your own pet name for him."

"You call him 'Olly.'"

"Everyone calls him that."

"You and his mother."

Gransen made a trifling gesture with his hand. "So, you and *Nev*. I'm trying to remember the last time I saw you be so chipper. Coincidence?" He blinked earnestly at her baleful look.

"I'm here because of what happened at the café. I had to."

Gransen peered at her, head tilting from side to side. "Did you?"

"My roof *fell* on him," Eunny said, incredulous. "He could've lost his job because of—"

"I know, I know, you're doing him a favor. Olly, my awkward little bean."

She scoffed. "Nothing little about him."

He immediately leaned forward. "How would you know?"

"I meant he's tall." Her shoulders hunched up around her ears. "Don't talk to me."

"Sure you did." Gransen sighed dramatically. "Everyone rides in on a white horse to help a *friend*."

"He got hurt helping *me*. Come on, Granse, you know that." Eunny gestured at the couch bed Ollas was relegated to sleeping upon and the end table with the salve and bandages— though they hadn't been needed as much of late. "I couldn't be the reason he had to give up something else," she murmured, trying for a wry smile. It felt more like a sad grimace.

Gransen sobered, continuing in a softer tone, "I think he's really glad you came up here. Grateful, even. Your friendship was—"

"He shouldn't be." She looked down at the table. "I'm like a bad luck charm. That's nothing to be grateful for."

"He doesn't blame you. You *do* know that, right? Olly would never—"

"He should," Eunny cut in, voice harsh. "And if he can't hold me accountable, then maybe it's for the best that I do. I've done nothing to deserve his gratitude."

Her magic being dragged out from under her, tearing away even as she tried so desperately to yank it back. How it had seared across Ollas, the crackling energy beneath her fingertips as his body writhed.

"I can never make it up to him, what I did," Eunny whispered. "Can't you see that?"

Gransen said nothing, mouth twisting as he considered her words.

She set her book aside and grabbed her cloak. "Good talk, but I'm going out for a bit."

"Eun." Gransen's voice had her pause at the door. "Your feelings are your feelings. I respect that. But Ollas doesn't blame you, and *you* should accept that, too. If you let yourself unclench for a minute, you'll realize it. Give him a chance."

"A chance to what?"

Gransen gave her a look. Eunny returned it.

"Are you going to make me say it?" he said, exasperated. "Because I will."

Ollas, with his freckles and his enthusiasm for gardening, which she'd always taken for nerdiness but which was also, unsettlingly, compelling. Those shy smiles when she teased him. Ollas, so happy that she was around. She'd realized it, subconsciously at the very least. Enjoyed it, too—that warm little sense of satisfaction she got at his attention, that *pleasure*. Eunny wouldn't admit it, but she was beginning to crave those feelings. Wanted to give them a chance to grow, to flourish, to see where they led. Wanted to take Ollas's forgiveness and run with it.

The solemnity was long gone from Gransen's face, a smug grin spreading from ear to ear.

"No." She left.

Disgruntled, Eunny wandered along the path through the greenhouse complex, eventually ducking into an empty Trunk when the constant drizzle grew to a downpour. She could always haul in some more bags of the water-retention amendment the elective was using. The spellwork to keep even moisture levels was fragile, and had a tendency to break down if it didn't like the precise ratios of imbued amendments or arcane work the students were testing.

Alongside the elective, Eunny had her own tray for an allotment of the same seeds the course used. Better to learn with the same materials, she told Ollas, since if she'd been an actual student she'd have lacked the prerequisites to even get through the door. It would be hard enough trying to mimic the students' work without trying to devise a new experiment.

Even at the small scale of a single elective, the sheer volume at which they trialed seeds with abandon was astounding to her. Ollas hadn't been kidding when he'd said there'd be a lot of failures and false starts. The students planted flat after flat, only to have their seeds sprout and die. In the beginning, the whole sad cycle happened within the same day. It had taken nearly two weeks before the seedlings started to last overnight. Another four days before they'd finally struck a promising mix that achieved faster, stable budding.

Reaching for the Trunk's wheelbarrow, Eunny paused as her eye caught on a new tray in the greenhouse's second antechamber. She went inside, crouching down beneath the rows of overflow plants and cuttings. A big philodendron had been scooted to the side to make space for a small tray only large enough to hold a pair of starter pots. Each held a small clump, no more than two or three stems of a nondescript, grass-like plant.

A flare in the back of Eunny's mind was followed by a flurry of twitches in her eye. She swore, jerking back from the low shelf, and stood, leaning against the upper rack for support. *Why* would those things be in here?

Ollas's mumbling to himself about having planted the overgrown patch on purpose, of needing to check...something. Innocent sounding words, but an irrational sense of dread settled in the pit of her stomach as she stared at the freshly propagated plants.

A knock on the antechamber's door drew her attention. Zhenya stood on the other side, visible through the window dominating the upper half of the door.

"Hey, Eunny," Zhenya called, her voice muffled by the glass. "Everything all right?"

"Yeah, just...headache." Understatement.

Grateful for an excuse to escape, Eunny went into the greenhouse's main room, where Zhenya had gathered small bags of different amendments and other materials into a stack of flat trays.

"What's all this for?" Eunny asked, reaching out to steady a piece of burlap Zhenya had tried to balance atop her load.

"The elective," Zhenya said. "Trying to prolong the corruption in the soil samples."

"Not something you hear every day, even at Sylveren."

It remained a mystery to the world how the Eyllic Empire had crafted its poison with so singular a purpose as to only cause destruction in the kingdom of Rhell. It seeped ever downward from where it had first been unleashed at Rhell's northeastern border, unrelenting in its pursuit of the magical wellspring in the capital city. Outward spread occurred more from measures taken trying to slow its progress than the poison naturally sprawling out. But once contaminated soil was taken down into the Valley—the only region willing to allow such a thing—it was quickly rendered inert. Whether it was the natural protection of the Valley itself, through the grace of its own wellspring or the lingering presence of its divine aspect, the Child, or something innate in the magical engineering of the poison, it didn't take hold beyond Rhell. Through careful handling and prodigious use of enchanted enclosures, mages at

Sylveren were able to maintain the blight in soil samples brought to the university for testing, but even those went sterile within weeks.

A new wrinkle for the elective arose when a shipment of soil from one of the Rhellian containment zones arrived completely inert. Despite having more concentrated levels of poison in the areas where restoration efforts had succeeded in curbing the spread, the poison rendered itself useless as soon as it entered the Valley. Great for border security, but a problem for Ollas and Rai's class and their baby seedlings.

Eunny took half of the load, throwing up an elbow to block Zhenya when she tried to reclaim it. "Hush. You're not going to be able to see over the top of this."

Zhenya relented with a smile. "Thanks." She rifled through a drawer, pulling out a few more random bottles before leading the way back to the Sapling, the mid-level greenhouse. "You don't need to stay. I just wanted to say hi."

"It's no trouble. Unless you want me to leave you alone," Eunny said, helping to unpack Zhenya's haul.

"Not at all. How are you liking grovetending?" Zhenya asked as she drew an ink bottle toward her and pulled a dip pen from her pocket. "I don't get to be in the lab as much as I'd hoped for the elective."

"You're already in there or class or the library often enough." Eunny let her eyes travel across the tidy rows of the students' trays lining one antechamber. "The gardening stuff is fine, but I don't think I've found my second calling."

She watched as Zhenya summoned a spot of golden-white light to the tip of her index finger and touched her pen's nib. A faint glow surrounded the point as she gave it a gentle swirl in the ink.

"This probably wasn't the best introduction," Zhenya said

as she began to inscribe runes on an empty glass jug's blank label. "Blended Growing is fun, or maybe Augmentation in Food Safety. That one keeps you on your toes with all the things catching fire or exploding. Can be smelly, though."

Eunny hummed in consideration. "What's this for?"

"Sealing enchantments. We're trying different methods of creating a biome for transporting the containment zone soil here."

"Ink works like that?"

Zhenya shrugged. "Within reason, we hope. If you want significant long-term storage, you're going to want real frost charms and collaborative work, but the contaminated soil was too reactive to the heavier duty spells. Ollas is looking better," she added, eyes on her work.

"Yea," Eunny agreed, a melancholic sigh rising from her chest. Goddess break, that feeling again. She forced a smile. "He's moving along pretty well. Pretty soon, he won't need me at all."

"We can't convince you to stay?" Zhen glanced sideways at her. "It's nice having you up here."

Eunny's smile was no longer forced, but the melancholy remained, only changing in tenor. "You're not rid of me just yet."

But her usefulness was running short. Eunny had always known it would, that helping Ollas was never meant to last more than a few weeks. She hadn't considered that she'd ever want to stay, though, and the prospect was growing ever so tempting.

But...she couldn't. She'd been serious when she'd said this was just to help out a friend, to make up for some of the harm she'd caused, that was all. No putting down roots in the community, no getting used to this path in her life. It wouldn't last. It couldn't.

Once Zhenya was finished, Eunny helped her carry her imbued glassware to the specialty greenhouse that housed the work of high-level mages. They parted ways, Zhenya going off to finish recordkeeping for Professor Rai. Eunny continued on toward the Grove, pausing at the foot of the outer stair. The energetic clamor of the Heartwood wafted toward her on the air, plucking at her chest. The sounds were blurred through the wood, but there was a joyous note to them, a warmth that invited with open arms.

Eunny made it halfway up the steps to the residence branch before stopping. She wasn't staying; she just already happened to be here, for the time being. If her days in the Grove were already numbered, what could it hurt to pass through the common room?

Eunny turned around and descended the stairs with measured steps. She'd do a quick pass through the common room, see if she could snag whatever the latest baked good was, maybe raid the tea stash, since she'd only brought one tin with her and some variety would be nice.

A dozen Grove residents of varying years were spread throughout the Heartwood. Several were engaged in a board game Eunny didn't recognize. Judging by the laughter and trio of flagons on the table, two of which were tipped on their sides, the logic of the game was a thing of the past. The cloying scent of cheap cordial fermented to within an inch of its life assailed her nose. Hard to say if it had been *enhanced* by magic or the limits of a student's budget. Probably both, and they'd pay for it with killer hangovers in the morning.

One of the smaller tables in the back had a nearly empty plate of cookies that looked like they couldn't decide if they were gray or purple.

"Careful," a voice murmured from Eunny's left. "Soph didn't get the proportions right." Ennis, the know-it-all kid from the elective, strolled over from their place on a nearby couch. "The dumplings were better." They pointed at a smaller, woefully empty plate.

Eunny broke off a corner of a cookie and nibbled. It smelled overwhelmingly of lavender and tasted like medicine that badly wanted to be soap. Maybe being alone in her room wasn't such a bad option after all. She went to the counter to peruse the tea selection. Ennis followed.

"You're not a grovetender," they said, helping themselves to a mug.

"You noticed."

"How'd you manage living here, then?"

"Friends in high places." Eunny helped herself to a disposable tea bag and opened a tin of a toasted green variety her aunt brought in from one of the Radiant Isles.

"You're a light mage. And you're old. Shouldn't you be in Belle or something?" The kid pulled three jars toward them and started spooning tiny dried pieces of bitter melon into a strainer basket in the mug.

"I'm working on—" Eunny eyed the amounts going into the mug. "What are you doing?"

"Making a wellness and digestion blend. What?" They gave her a defensive look. "I read up about it."

Eunny pressed her eyes closed. For patience, and also to block out the image of the kid adding heaps of blaze-spotted gentian to their mug. The clink of the spoon against a jar of powdered dandelion made Eunny fling her hand out to stop Ennis from lifting the lid.

"You need about four more stomachs to manage any of that."

"There's a chapter on this in the Basics to Herbalism book," Ennis said, a mulish jut to their chin.

"Ever heard of a thing called moderation?" Not to mention

that the student-run mercantile had an entire section devoted to herbal remedies. Blends that were made under the supervision of Magister levels, not two lines in an introductory textbook.

"It's good for me." Ennis shook one of the jars. "Extra goodness."

Gods all break.

"Maybe if you were part ruminant." Eunny knocked their hand away and emptied the strainer into the compost bin, shushing Ennis's indignant squawk. "I've known you for all of a day and I can tell you don't need that much cooling. Move."

Eunny swept the kid aside, dumping their disaster mug and exchanging their jars for a mild tisane of forest herbs with speckled ashberries for interest.

Adding enough hot water to fill the mug, she warned, "Don't touch that until I'm done," before grabbing another teabag. Taking her time, Eunny made herself another blend, raiding the tins of frosted chamomile and dried elderberries.

Ennis huffed, loudly, but did as they were ordered. When Eunny finally gave them a nod, they slowly lifted the mug. Much sniffing and suspicious looks were done, but when they finally deigned to take a tiny sip, it was quickly followed by a larger one.

"It's fine," they sniffed. "Could use more honey."

"Rot your teeth out." Eunny slid the pot in their direction before grabbing her pilfered teabags. "If you really want something for your gut, just go to the student store. Get the free ones and sweeten back here."

Ennis rolled their eyes as they took another sip. "Okay, Mom." They smirked at Eunny's appalled look, considering the mug. "Guess you know something." They sauntered back to the couch.

Eunny shook her head. It wasn't even apothecary work so

much as using some common sense. Besides, she didn't do that work anymore. This did nothing to change her mind about that.

She snorted, covering her mouth to suppress the laugh that bubbled up. The begrudging concession *did* make her feel an obnoxious amount of vindication.

"Hey, Handywoman Song!" Ennis called, waving at her from their spot on the couch.

Eunny wandered over. "Handywoman?"

"It's what you are, isn't it?" The kid shrugged. "If you studied body magic when you were here, how'd you get so good at repair work?"

"I love the repair café!" exclaimed a red-haired girl sitting next to Ennis who Eunny vaguely recognized from being around the Grove. "Will it open again soon? The Stitchery were teaching us decorative mending."

"I'm not sure. There was a lot of damage," Eunny said, feeling monstrous as the girl visibly wilted at the news. "You like it that much?"

"Yes! I didn't know how to do any of my own repairs before," the girl said.

Somehow, Eunny ended up seated on the couch, listening to the life story of the girl—the aforementioned Soph of the tragic cookies—and how she'd come to Sylveren after growing up in North District, Graelynd. It was strangely pleasant, hearing her exuberance for the repair café; Eunny had grown too used to Gransen's brand of obsession disguised as passion. She found herself sharing her tale of summers spent at the teashop and finally deciding to make the move permanent when life in Central no longer held any appeal. It was a truncated, glossed-over version of events, but the mixed emotions of fear and excitement at starting over were true enough.

Do you ever miss it? Your life there? No, no she didn't. But the life she'd hemmed herself into, a repair café and a profession devoid of magic—it was getting harder to remain content with that life, too. Harder not to be tempted to give other things a chance.

When Eunny finally left to meander back upstairs, a flicker of the regret she saw in Ennis and Soph's faces at the night coming to a close resonated with her own.

Chapter Ten

A FEW MORE DAYS PASSED, and though Gransen never broached the topic again, their conversation lingered at the back of Eunny's mind.

"Give him a chance."

"A chance to what?"

"Are you going to make me say it?"

Yet every time Eunny was around Ollas—schlepping his bags, dragging crates around, assisting with the watering—though conversation flowed easily between them, inertia kept the words inane.

Everything was so good right now. Uncomplicated. Ollas would get excited about some garden thing, and even though Eunny couldn't understand half of it, just listening to him had that satisfied warmth filling her brain. Eunny didn't think she'd been *unhappy* before, but there was something nice about laughing in the morning over breakfast, getting her hands dirty in the greenhouse most afternoons, hanging out in the Heartwood or even just in the apartment's main room each evening. Slapping the papers out of Gransen's hands whenever she got the chance. Joking with Ollas. Making him blush.

It had her thinking—not seriously, but just for fun, during her off hours—about what it could mean for her, accepting the notion of Ollas's forgiveness. Giving him a chance, as Gransen had said. But the old guilt rose up every time, and as she tidied up the living area one afternoon, she realized that Ollas's bottle of healing salve hadn't been used in a few days. Most of the bandages remained in a neat, untouched pile by his couch bed. They were nearing the month mark of her "assisting" him. No point in risking the good times they were having when soon she wouldn't be there at all.

But not quite yet.

Taking advantage of a rare break in the weather, Eunny went into town. She hurried past the repair café, where, barely visible in her periphery, boards and water-repellant fabric shades temporarily replaced the busted windows.

Stepping inside the Mighty Leaf, Eunny flashed the note she'd received from Yerina earlier that morning to her Uncle Dex. He gave her a gruff nod and jerked his head to indicate her favorite booth at the back. Considering gruffness was his resting state, Eunny almost wouldn't have read anything into it, but coupled with her aunt's note being devoid of her usual cheeriness, it had a sense of trepidation growing within Eunny as she made her way through the tearoom.

She saw her aunt first and waved to get Yerina's attention as she walked forward. Yerina quickly stood up, a nervous smile on her face.

"Eunny, thank you for coming. I'm sorry I didn't let you know sooner," Yerina said, coming toward her.

"It's no trouble. What's up, Auntie? You don't usually..." Eunny trailed off, her gaze going over her aunt's shoulder as she noticed the booth was still occupied. She'd know that immaculately twisted updo anywhere.

"Aunt Yerina..." Eunny whispered, exasperation in her tone.

"She wanted to meet with you, but she didn't think you'd come if she asked you herself," Yerina said, as if it was a reasonable explanation.

"Well, maybe Mother does know best sometimes, because she'd be right."

"Eunny," Yerina said softly, laying a hand on her arm. "She's come a long way."

Two visits in as many months—unheard of for Bioon after six years of nothing. Eunny would've been happy to maintain their distance. But Yerina's round face was full of silent pleading, of hope and heartbreak for this sad excuse for a family reunion. Eunny could return her mother's snubs with vicious pleasure, but disappointing her auntie?

Ensuring that her sigh was audible, Eunny gave her aunt a brief hug before dragging herself the few steps to the booth. She plopped onto the cushioned bench and reached for the teapot in the middle of the table, eyes following Yerina's retreat to the front of the tearoom.

"Eunji, so kind of you to join me," Bioon said.

"Making Auntie Yerina do your dirty work? Low, even for you."

"A sad day when I must stoop to such means because my own daughter can't be bothered otherwise to see me." Bioon's lips curled into a cold smile as she sipped her tea. "How is the elective going?"

"Don't your superiors get the reports? Or do you have apprentices do the trivial work?"

"I'm asking you," Bioon said. "You're an outside observer. A unique perspective, as dear Ollas so nicely put it."

Hearing his name from her mother's mouth made Eunny's skin crawl. "The elective seems fine. The plants are lasting more than a day. Rai and Ollas seem happy with the progress."

Bioon made a noncommittal noise. A few moments of

silence passed as they regarded each other over their tea. Eunny broke it first. Better to get these ridiculous games over and done with than sit here for an hour, going in circles.

"What do you really want?" Eunny asked. "I have things I could be doing back at the school if you're just going to waste time."

"You've become so crass, daughter." Bioon's tone was light, almost playfully reproachful, but her gaze was sharp as ever. She set the teacup aside. "You're trained to recognize the value of the product this exploratory class is working on. Something you should be able to ascertain even without your magic."

"Was there a question in that?"

"Are they getting close to having something worth sending to us?"

Eunny scoffed. "You've gotten the reports. I know because I saw Ollas write at least two of them." She pasted a sweet smile onto her face. "You should come to the greenhouse and observe."

"Perhaps I will," Bioon said, matching Eunny's fake smile. "The reports are a condition of the Coalition's sponsorship— they present the information in a most favorable light. I'm asking you for the unvarnished truth."

"I'm not a grovetender, remember. Whatever Ollas and Rai have told you is more than I'm going to know. They wouldn't lie."

"Omission," Bioon murmured. "There haven't been any additions to the elective's trials? No new seed variants or base materials aside from the original outline?"

Eunny could feel her face screwing up in confusion. "No? My understanding is that asking for two hybrids in one term was already next to impossible. Why do you think they'd add even more?"

Bioon's shoulders lifted in a dainty shrug. "We're a month

in, with nothing to show for it. Such failure brings priorities into—"

"A priority aside from helping with the poison? Helping Rhell?" Eunny raised her eyebrows in mild exasperation. "Don't confuse Sylveren for the Coalition, Mother. We actually have morals."

For a moment, Bioon said nothing, eyes roving over Eunny's face. Then she smiled again, a small twist of her mouth that was more smirk than anything else. "It's my job to ask, Eunji."

"You know, the Restorers are backing the work done in the elective," Eunny said. "Maybe you should put some more faith in that."

Bioon clasped her hands together. "The Coalition protects trade interests, Eunji. We're not in the business of cultivating unfounded hope."

"Unfounded?" Incredulity colored her voice. "There's been real progress made at Sylveren, just in the last *year*. Since all you care about is money, ever consider the health of trade if you'd all gotten off your asses and—"

"Progress? Is that what you think they've achieved in Rhell?" The disdain in her mother's voice was so thick Eunny almost thought she could feel it. "One tiny step forward and they've hit a wall. Now the Restorers must allocate resources to fix what your *progress* has wrought."

"Didn't stop the Coalition from jumping in for their cut," Eunny shot back. "If it's so useless, why bother 'allocating resources?'"

Bioon scoffed, but Eunny had the measure of her. The Coalition would fuss, but gods all break if the elective was successful and they were left out.

"It's contained," Eunny said. "That's more than anyone's done since the war started."

"The first bioremediation class that was supposed to stem

from the Rhell Accord was to grow something that could actually rejuvenate the ground. Instead, you are spending an entire academic term on reactionary work. Only in the kindest of readings is this, at best, a lateral move. Many of my colleagues think it a waste."

"Then it's a good thing we're in the Valley, where people think responsibly and not with their purse strings," Eunny spat. "Easy for you to scorn. People are working themselves to the bone here. What've you ever done for Graelynd except for bully folk into shit trade agreements?"

"You still think like a child," Bioon said, dismissing Eunny's words with a wave of her hand. "A nation as powerful as Graelynd has duties that extend beyond itself. Your precious Valley is alone up here and thinks in those same narrow terms."

"Didn't stop your precious Coalition from asking them to host that travesty of a trade delegation." Bitterness made Eunny's lip curl. "Didn't stop them from inserting themselves into the elective."

"An insertion we're paying for." Bioon folded her hands together, giving Eunny a considering look. "Do you think about the delegation?"

"Nope," Eunny said, popping the 'p' just to watch her mother wince. "Why?"

"You don't recall the trade talks?"

"You mean the private tent talks I was excluded from? I don't like to think about the worst day of my life, and when I do, I remember that it was your fault I was there."

"I'm flattered you think I have the power to disrupt negotiations between countries," Bioon said in a dry tone, "but I didn't cause your problem with your magic, Eunji."

Maybe not directly, but Bioon was the one who'd dragged Eunny from her Adept Two studies to accompany her at the delegation. Claimed a mender's knowledge and skills would be useful, though Eunny suspected her mother had been more interested in having a young, Sylveren-educated Graelynder along for the optics back home in Central. Maybe she'd thought having a younger person around would remind people to keep the talks civil. Either way, it hadn't worked. Eunny's presence hadn't stopped the Eyllics from implementing their hostile takeover, sneaking in a dozen more guards than had been allotted in the delegation's terms.

"We're done here," Eunny said. "Either accept the reports Ollas is sending or, next time, check the greenhouse yourself. Don't make Auntie Yerina cover for you."

"Actually, Eunji, I'd appreciate an accounting from you as well." Bioon raised a hand when Eunny started to argue. "I will, of course, continue to defer to Ollas and Professor Rai, but I'm interested in your thoughts as well. The work that goes into assisting, in your own words. I'm sure you're seeing things from a different angle from the regular students."

Reflex had a nasty retort on the tip of Eunny's tongue, a barb about not being at the beck and call of the Coalition or her mother. A tingle of instinct at the back of her mind gave Eunny pause. Something about her mother's intent gaze, the too-casual way in which she'd voiced her request, aroused a tendril of suspicion that Eunny couldn't immediately place. She wasn't as good at playing games as her mother—just one of the consequences of having a heart—but Eunny had been frustrated by the woman and her misdirection enough times that she could recognize some of the tells.

"I'm not going to be around much longer anyway," Eunny said. "Ollas is about ready to manage on his own."

She watched the interest drop away from her mother's face, whatever value Eunny might've had diminishing at her statement.

"How wonderful for him." Bioon slipped from the booth,

swishing her cloak about her shoulders. She looked down at her daughter, an imperious tilt to her head. It was a familiar look, and Eunny hated that a part of herself was still mesmerized by it—repulsed, yet unable to look away. There was something coldly beautiful about her mother. Unfeeling, and the soft pieces that remained in Eunny yearned to know how she managed it.

"It doesn't surprise me that you've fit in so well here." Bioon spun on her heel and walked away, brushing past Yerina with a shake of her head.

Eunny followed at a slower pace. "That went well," she deadpanned to her aunt. "I'll come by again later."

She trudged back to the school, Bioon's probing words jangling in her ears. Her disdain was nothing new, but the veiled questions suggested something else. Eunny couldn't remember the last time a conversation with her mother *didn't* have at least an element of antagonism, but bringing up the delegation? Asking Eunny to report on Ollas?

Any way she looked at it, Eunny didn't like what she saw, but she didn't have anything concrete to validate her suspicions, either.

As she meandered up the path to the Grove, she scanned each of the greenhouse buildings she passed. A few Adept-levels working in Sapling, but no Ollas. Eunny turned toward the main tree. Movement in her periphery had her spinning around in time to see Ollas's back disappearing through the door at Trunk.

Changing course, Eunny followed him.

Chapter Eleven

PEEKING through the window set into Trunk's outer door, Eunny saw that Ollas was alone. She sauntered in, a mock disapproving look on her face. "I thought you were grading?"

Ollas glanced over his shoulder, a smile lighting his face, and pointed to a short pile of paperwork. "I did." He hunched his shoulders sheepishly. "I'm just taking a break."

She stopped next to him, boosting herself up so she could sit on the countertop, legs dangling. "Slacking off, I see," she joked, though she had to force levity into her tone and smooth the tightness from her expression.

Ollas peered at her. "Problem at the Mighty Leaf?"

Eunny scrunched her face in displeasure. "Just...mother problems. Nothing new, it's just been a while." She tilted her head as she eyed the topmost paper. "The novices going to be all tears after their first university exam?"

"I'm sure this wasn't their first," Ollas said. "Jolly has the Intro to Arcane Influences on Statistics class this term, and she likes to nip in the bud any thoughts that her name and personality are related by giving an 'evaluation quiz' the first week."

Eunny winced, shaking her head. "Hang on." She turned the paper so it faced her. "Are you changing the answer key?"

"Yes. Half of the class has gotten that question wrong." Ollas's mouth curved with a soft smile.

Eunny stared at him. "And? Tell them to study harder."

"Half of the class, Eunny," Ollas repeated. "I strike any question with that kind of failure rate for lack of clarity."

"Isn't that being soft on them?" Eunny folded her arms over her chest. "Life isn't going to give them a pass for not understanding the question. You're not doing them any favors with coddling, and I don't just mean if they go to mean old Central. This won't pass in Sylvan, either."

"A majority failure rate is indicative of a larger problem," Ollas said, his voice patient but firm, without condescension. "Either it's a failure in my teaching of the subject or a failure in how I've worded the question. Either way, it's a failure on my part."

Eunny squinted at him. "What about the ones who got it right? Extra credit? Tough luck?"

Ollas chuckled. "The question is struck for everyone."

"So they get nothing for getting it right the first time around."

"The point is more to educate the whole as evenly as I can." His smile turned wry. "It's not a perfect approach."

"I'll say," Eunny scoffed, though she was more flummoxed than disdainful. "I'm still convinced my Intro to Herbalism professor wrote his tests as opaquely as possible so he could yell at our miserable scores and turn it into a lecture about detail and intuition and 'your excuses don't mean anything to your patient if they're dead, Miss Song.'"

Ollas tilted his head toward her. "You think I'm a soft-hearted progressive turning out a weakened generation of emotionally fragile would-be scholars." Though he tried to keep his tone neutral, amusement crept in.

"That was specific. I take it Admin hasn't always approved?"

"There have been discussions, but no one's come for my head yet."

Eunny laughed. "I'll give you that your approach is a damn sight nicer than what we got at the House of Healing, but maybe body magic needs to be more exacting. People get touchy about pain, who'd have thought? Or I'm just bitter. Possessing empathy and expressing it... Eh. Not the same."

"You're plenty empathetic."

Eunny rolled her eyes. "No wonder your students love you."

"I get my share of bad reviews." Ollas grinned. "But you didn't come here for my thoughts on pedagogy."

She shrugged, gaze roving around the greenhouse before settling on the rear antechamber's door, which reminded her of the trayful of baby plants she'd found a few days before. She glanced sidelong at him, eyebrows rising. "You started another project without telling me."

"Project?" A furrow marred his brow, then recognition hit. "Oh, the divisions. Yes, come see."

Ollas hopped down from the counter. He grabbed the potting tray he'd been assembling before she came in and beckoned for Eunny to follow him into the antechamber.

"Isn't it my job to help with your stuff?" she asked.

"I can manage a few steps," he said with mock indignation.

Eunny poked him. "Your arm's moving pretty well, too. You don't really need me at all."

"I need you," Ollas blurted out. His hand came up, stuttering in the air as if he couldn't decide whether to press his fist to his mouth or make some other gesture. He settled for an exaggerated roll of his recovering shoulder. "I still need you for the overhead lifting."

The pleased feeling was back, fluttering giddily in her chest. Eunny pinched her lips together to keep from grinning from ear to ear like a fool. "Sure, we'll go with that."

She squatted next to the seed tray, careful not to touch anything. Just her luck that she hadn't thought to bring her gloves. The faint pulling sensation was back, but not nearly as intense as the night she'd fallen into the outside patch. It was more of a hum, vibrating unobtrusively at the back of her mind, waiting.

"I've been looking into the origin of the plants outside. They're from the delegation." Ollas cleared space on the rack's upper shelf so Eunny could place the seed tray on top. He glanced at her, apprehension crossing his face. "Are you— We don't have to work on—"

"It's fine," Eunny said with a casual shake of her head. "How'd you get your hands on these?"

"The Sentinels confiscated everything at the camp at the time. These were just seeds back then, deemed mundane. The record log was incomplete, so I'm still trying to hunt down the notes we took when they were first brought in, but I remember Rai and some of the Sentinels' mages testing them."

"If they're not magical, why are you fussing with them now?"

Ollas caressed a leaf with one hand. "They're... changing. See how the leaf blade is widening? They're developing distinct petioles."

Eunny squinted. "Meaning?"

He chuckled. "They're looking more like this"—he tapped the philodendron next to them—"and less like grass."

"And that's rare?" she guessed.

"Very. And they feel... It's almost like I can—" A spark of

golden light flickered at the tip of his index finger. One little spark that fizzled as quickly as it had appeared. Ollas huffed to himself, as if this was a common occurrence. "It's like they want magic, but they don't react to it. Not that I can give them much, so I'm going with the next best thing." He nodded toward the potting tray and the variety of soil mixes and amendments he'd gathered.

"You have an entire patch of them outside," Eunny said, a reluctant, resigned feeling settling into her bones. "Why are you making more?"

"There's something about them," Ollas said, excitement in his face. "The delegation had them for a reason. I want to run some tests to see if I can figure out why."

"Fine, I'm game," Eunny sighed. "Can I wear your gloves? I forgot mine."

He slapped his pair into her hand. "I just want to amend the current transplant mix."

She picked up a small scoop. "Okay, if you handle the plants, I'll shovel."

They set to work. Eunny spooned different amendments into the tray at Ollas's prompting, mixing it with a hand rake as he fluffed the dirt around the fresh divisions of the delegation plants.

"Do you, uh…" Ollas began in a hesitant voice. When Eunny gestured for him to continue, he said, "Do you remember plants like these at the delegation?"

"No, they only had me check dried herbs and some seeds the Eyllics were offering," Eunny said, pausing as she closed her eyes in thought. "Remedies for aid workers and trade merchants to use while making deliveries in Rhell. Supposed to be a goodwill gesture, but…"

Eunny opened her eyes so she could deposit the mixture

into the pots. "Nothing we hadn't already seen, from what I could tell. I think most of them were just for show—"

A puff of dust swirled up. As she reached for the watering can, Eunny started to sneeze, accidentally taking a step toward Ollas and brushing against the plant's closest leaf. A blur of hot and cold emanated from the dirt mix, the churn of magic unmistakable as it filtered straight through her clothing like the barrier wasn't there. It caught her by surprise, the increasingly familiar *pulling* at her mind. At her center. A swirl of magic flowed through her fingers, a sympathetic vibration humming beneath her skin. The reaction was subconscious. Second nature, even after all this time.

Even if she'd abandoned it. Called her magic lost. Called— *believed*—it dead to her. But her spark caught in the arcane reaction happening in the seed tray and swept her along. The flow of magic was so reminiscent, just for a second, of how it had felt on that awful day. Wild, rushing, draining away from her.

No. Eunny fought panic. She was here, in the greenhouse. Not in the delegation's camp. But the magic was swirling through her fingers, frissons of cold energy pricking her skin. She remembered slipping. Falling. Feeling like some vital part of her was being sucked out. She was losing control, *again.* A scream built in the back of her throat.

"Keep stirring."

Eunny blinked. She knew that voice.

"Sorry, should've mentioned the reaction. Stir, stir, stir," Ollas said, making an encouraging motion with his hands. "The enchantment in the amendment weakens if it gets hot or cold spots."

Automatically, she moved her rake through the dirt, sloshing water onto the dusty mix. The motion dispersed some of the tingling sensation. She focused on the sound of Ollas's calm voice, willing her hands not to shake.

"It'll even out as it sets, and the spell in the granules helps ward against rot. Not perfectly, but they help with the water retention worked into the mix and the cold spells." Ollas added more dirt to the tray and gently tamped it around the base of the plantlets. "Lets us push it with how wet we can let the trays get in this climate. Especially these days."

Eunny kept dragging the hand tool through the dirt until the roar of blood no longer rushed through her ears. Her hand only shook a little as she set the rake aside. She stared at the plants. The pulling sensation was dissipating, the arcane flow sinking into the dirt. Fading. No, *absorbing*. With her panic easing, Eunny realized that the magic reaction wasn't the same as when she'd lost control. That had been a terrifying, frictionless drain as her magic streamed away. But these plants, or the dirt, or some combination thereof, they didn't pull her magic away so much as absorb what was at hand.

That pulling sensation. Its familiarity went beyond her fall into the patch outside the greenhouse. These seemingly benign plants, leftovers from the delegation... She was certain she'd never seen them, at least not in this fully grown form. But the absorptive properties...

A vague memory flitted in the foggy recesses of her mind, of times she'd tried so hard to never think of again.

"Eunji, come look at these. They say they're healing plants."

"What do you expect me to do with these?" Eunny held the seeds up in front of her face. *"Goddess break, Mother! For the last time, if you wanted plant knowledge, you should've brought a grovetender. Or a mender who gardened. Anyone but me!"*

She'd probed the seeds with her magic, for all the good it would do. Unless they were meant to be eaten, Eunny wasn't the kind of apothecary who grew her own wares, and thus didn't know what to do when given plants before they even started to become plants. The seeds hadn't reacted at all, just sucked up her magic. No resonance, no spark, no indication that they were anything useful. They were just there, taking up space. Which was rather how Eunny had felt at the delegation.

Maybe Ollas was right—something was going on. With the plants, and with her mother. It was too coincidental. Eunny could accept that the Coalition would want to keep an eye on the elective given its obsession with being in everyone's business when it came to trade. But the strange magnetism of the plants, and how that magnetism seemed to be affecting not just her but Ollas, too? Bioon repeatedly asking Eunny about new developments in the elective, wanting Eunny to spy on Ollas? It didn't make sense. She didn't understand it.

But...she didn't have to. If Ollas's plant nerdery was going to put him in the path of the Coalition, of her mother, Eunny knew whose side she would take every time.

"You said you were looking into the records for these things?" Eunny asked, waving a hand at the tray as Ollas resettled it on the lower shelf. "Let me know if I can do anything. I need plausible reasons to be helping you with your work."

After they'd cleaned up from their adventures in the greenhouse, Ollas grabbed his exam paperwork and motioned toward the door. "Home?"

A heady warmth filled him when she nodded. It was a simple affirmation, and likely one he was taking too literally, but having Eunny consider the apartment her home...it was a feeling he never wanted to lose.

Eunny fell into step beside him.

"Did you feel anything?" she asked as they locked up. "Anything weird? When I was adding the new dirt."

"Soil." Ollas dodged her swatting hand. "A little."

Eunny stilled.

"But I'm so used to it at this point I don't really notice. I should've warned you. Sorry about that." He gave her an abashed smile.

"You mean, the...?" Eunny trailed off, confused.

"The imbued amendments. Even mundanes can feel the physical aspects of the spells when they're activated," Ollas explained. "I forgot that it can be surprising if you're not expecting it. These cold pellets have a bite."

"Yeah, that—that was a shock."

They lapsed into silence, but one that lacked their usual easy comfort. When Ollas chanced a look out the corner of his eye, Eunny appeared pensive, chewing at her lower lip.

"Did something happen tonight?" he asked, voice soft. "You seemed a little upset when you came in."

Eunny made a series of annoyed sounds as they took the lift up to their apartment, finally muttering, "No. Just Bioon being herself. Thinks she's the sword of Graelynd or something, the way she went on about national pride bullshit. Shame on me for slumming it up here in my *precious Valley*." Her tone turned sour for the last words.

Kicking off her shoes, she dropped onto his couch bed instead of seeking her room. "I think I hate her, Nev." She fell back, addressing the ceiling: "I hate my mother, and that probably makes me a bad person, and you know what? I don't even feel bad about it."

Ollas looked around, but the apartment was otherwise empty. He sat on the edge of the couch, unsure of how to respond.

Eunny's cheeks puffed as she blew out a long breath. "I

think the worst part is how Aunt Yerina still tries. Thinks we can be a happy family. She doesn't *say it*, but I know she's disappointed in me for not trying more."

"I'm sure that's not true."

Eunny huffed softly to herself, the sound stretching into a yawn. "Gods, I'm tired. She sucks the life out of me."

"I'd take you as a protector of the Valley any day over your ma as the champion of Graelynd."

Eunny huffed a laugh. She plucked at the edges of the blanket, briefly meeting his eyes before looking back up at the ceiling. "How'd you escape all this?"

"Which part?"

"The expectations. I mean, your mom's great and all, but she never put any demands on you? Ever?" Her eyes drifted closed.

Ollas fiddled with his own corner of the blanket. "Well, she's hinted that she'd like grandchildren someday."

Eunny smiled, eyes still shut. "Why hasn't that worked out? You're the Homegrown Hero." She didn't see his grimace. "You're really going to tell me that didn't get you any fans, wanted or otherwise?"

Ollas felt heat rise in his cheeks. Glad that she wasn't watching him, he murmured, "Nothing serious."

"Never had a thing with Zhen? Before she got all obsessed with that dickbag from—"

"Rhydian's not so bad. It's complicated."

"Is that Sentinels brotherhood I hear?" Eunny cracked one eye to give him an unamused look before closing it again. "You sound like her. But that proves my point. Nothing with Zhen? Before you guys decided to just be friends."

Ollas winced. His ma had asked the same thing a time or two. Probably most of the upper levels in the Grove had wondered the same. "No, just friends. Good ones, but only that. People used to tease her about it, until you put a stop to that."

"Kids are jerks."

"And you put the fear of the Goddess in them. Made believers out of me and Zhen, that's for sure."

Eunny yawned, spreading her arms wide. "That's right. Worship at the Altar of Song."

"I think I always have," Ollas murmured, more to himself than to her. He forced a grin. "Did Zhen ever tell you about how she confirmed our friendship?"

Eunny shook her head, her drowsy "uh-uh" muffled behind closed lips.

"She must've been twelve, and I was about to turn fifteen. And she was so shy about it—but direct, you know how she is when something's bothering her." Ollas smiled to himself. He recounted the tale of a young, nervous, but determined Zhenya practically cornering an only somewhat older, equally nervous Ollas in the library and blurting out that she liked being friends, only friends, and was that okay. Gods, and the relief they'd both felt to know they were on the same page.

He glanced at Eunny, noting the way her face had softened, her stillness only disturbed by slow, even breaths.

"I like Zhen, but..." Ollas spoke softly, his confession barely more than a whisper. Lost to sleep, Eunny didn't hear him. He carefully got up and tucked the blanket around her shoulders. She didn't so much as stir.

"It never would've worked," he murmured. "She isn't you."

With quiet steps, Ollas went back to the table to finish his grading.

Chapter Twelve

It had to be obvious to anyone who saw him that Ollas didn't need her assistance anymore. He got around well now, no longer needing his cane. His limp only became pronounced late in the day, and even then, only if he'd been rushing back and forth between his office and the greenhouse several times. Which should've been part of Eunny's job, except he went out of his way not to ask. But he didn't mention her role as his helper becoming obsolete, so neither did she. The arrangement was always meant to be temporary. Whenever the end came, she'd accept it. Hopefully, with grace. Regardless, she wouldn't be seeking it out, either.

By the end of the week, Ollas's secret plant project showed a marked difference due to his experimenting. The leaves had all converted to their more traditional leaf shape, whereas the overgrown patch outside still mostly resembled grass. He and Eunny had scoured the greenhouse records for any reports that might shed light on the provenance of the plants, but had come up short. Annoyingly short, according to Ollas. Unreasonably so.

"We have documentation, I know it," he'd said after they'd

spent an afternoon poring over old ledgers but had found nothing aside from a short entry from when he'd first started the seeds. "Earthen take me, I swear I remember logging more than this."

Pointing out that maybe his memory had become a little hazy in the six years that had passed didn't change Ollas's mind. Which left the Sentinels' records as their last option, and Eunny couldn't help with that. With midterms approaching, their search for the missing records was put on hold.

But, though she'd been reluctant to get involved, Eunny couldn't deny that the nebulous "feeling" Ollas spoke of when it came to the plants; she felt it, too. A sense of being drawn in. Called to, but in a way she couldn't accurately describe. With growing frequency, she found herself stealing into the greenhouse during Ollas's office hours to check on the two little pots stashed away on the bottom shelf, or peeking through the window at the patch outside.

Which was how she found herself there one rainy afternoon, slipping into the greenhouse as rain lashed the windowpanes. Eunny chanced a look around, but Trunk was empty, per usual. She donned gloves, though that was more for her own false sense of security—she suspected that the plants' unnamed pull defied physical barriers—then picked one of the secret pots up and set it on the rack's upper shelf.

Ollas had observed how the plants seemed to take up the magic in their substrate. They *wanted* it, but they put nothing out in response. No growth spurts or setting buds. No adverse reaction either, of rot or wilt or yellowing leaves. They were stubbornly steady in their continued existence.

But the pull remained. Took the form of a soft humming, both a sound and a sensation in her mind. It called to her in a way that had no right to feel so natural to someone who didn't have a lick of earth magic. True, all the arcane disciplines stemmed from light magic, but Eunny had never had an affinity for earth. In her old life as an apothecary, her magic had resonated with the body side, light magic tuned for healing. She was no elementalist, yet something emanated from the plants and drew her in, even though they remained as nondescript as ever, just with different leaves. No striking variegation, no glimmer or visible aura. They were simple and green.

Ignoring how silly she felt, Eunny let her eyes drift closed, focusing on the invisible pull. She followed it, trying to map the nature of it in her head, searching for anything recognizable. There was a familiar note to it, though she couldn't place how she'd have known. She delved deeper, gently pinching a leaf between her gloved fingers. Through the barrier of her leather glove, the pull evoked a restless curiosity that plucked at her memory. She'd felt it before, and not just the night she'd gone to convince Ollas to let her assist during his recovery. This feeling of certainty went beyond that. Had persisted for weeks, maybe a month. All summer long, but in a softer, vaguer sense. Building in momentum, or intensity, yet still incomplete. Something was missing, such that even as she stood here with the plant in her hands, Eunny couldn't make sense of the puzzle.

She didn't recognize how the pulling sensation grew to form a pulse until it was too late. Heat slithered across her skin as two pinpricks of golden light gathered on her fingertips. A startled jerk of her wrist shed them like water drops onto the dirt; one blink of her eyes and they were gone, absorbed into the surface. Eunny inwardly braced, ready for a flurry of eye twitches or for her magic to go berserk like the first time she'd encountered the plants.

She waited, heartbeat pounding at her throat.

Nothing happened. The tension left her shoulders as she breathed out in a shaky exhale. She glanced toward the antechamber door, but no one was around to witness her standing there like a fool.

Eunny replaced the pot on its lower shelf, and as she straightened, motion in her periphery caught her attention. Through the smudged greenhouse windows, she spied a pair of riders as they trotted toward the school's stable. She only saw them through a gap in the greenhouse complex's hedge, and then they were gone again.

It might only have been a glimpse, and at a distance, but she knew that dark-haired head, the indigo cloak.

She bolted for the door.

Eunny caught up as the couple was leaving the stable on foot.

"Dae!" she called, hurrying toward them.

The dark-haired woman turned, a smile already lighting her face before she'd even spotted the source of her name. "Eunny! What are you—"

The rest of the question cut off in an "oof" as Eunny launched herself at one of her best friends in the world, Anadae Helm.

"What are *you* doing here?" Eunny asked, recovering enough to hold Dae out at arm's length. "Are you sick? You're sick. Why haven't you said anything?"

Eunny searched her friend's face, but it gave nothing away. Sure, being of both Hanyeok and Graelynd descent, Dae's complexion was always a shade or two lighter than Eunny's own, but it had a healthy enough look. Her cheeks were a bit pink and wind-chapped, the dark circles under her eyes a bit pronounced. Her gait seemed a touch stiff, but if she'd arrived from Rhell then that meant over a week in the saddle, and Dae was no seasoned horsewoman. All valid excuses to look slightly ragged at the edges, except, perhaps, for their current direction. The path the trio had stopped on wasn't bound for the administrative area of the Dome or even the Towers, where elementalists like Dae and her partner, Ezzyn Sor'vahl, studied. Instead, they were on the road leading toward the House of Syvrine. There'd be no cause for two elementalists to head toward the domain of light magic unless—

"Goddess break. Are you…are you *sick*-sick?" Eunny fought the urge to reach for her magic and send it questing into her friend. At Dae's scoff, Eunny looked instead to the pale blond man standing beside her. "Sor'vahl?"

The Rhellian man's lips pinched together as he exchanged looks with Dae. "She needs to spend some time outside of Rhell."

"I do not. This is just—"

"Why?" Eunny narrowed her eyes, head flipping back and forth between the two. "It's the poison, isn't it? You have the sickness we've been—"

"I'm not— I don't have anything serious," Dae said.

"What have you been hearing?" Ezzyn demanded.

"That more people are getting sick from the containment." Eunny released Dae enough to loop their arms and begin towing her toward the Healing Hut. "It's all hush-hush. I only know about it because I'm helping with the elective the Restorers funded."

"You are?" Surprise tipped Dae's voice up.

"I'll explain later," Eunny said. "Why are you coming all the way back to the Valley? Couldn't you just take a break outside a contaminated zone?"

"Perhaps this should wait until we're somewhere more private," Ezzyn murmured, indicating a gaggle of Initiate level students walking toward them on their way to class. He glanced upward. "And dry."

Though the downpour had lessened to a drizzle, Eunny took his point, asking instead about their journey and how their work in Ezzyn's homeland of Rhell was going. Dae and Ezzyn had spent the summer making their way across the small kingdom, aiding the implementation of a new ward system to fight the poison that had continued spreading across Rhell in the six years since the Eyllic War had ended. Dae's Adept One research dovetailed with Ezzyn's Magister-level work, resulting in wards that could finally contain the spread instead of merely slow it.

The danger of the Eyllic-made poison was twofold: magical in nature, the poison had an ability to endure and return despite the strongest cleansing efforts made by the brightest minds throughout the Alliance of Empyrean Territories. Even worse, the poison fought back. It drained all who came into contact with it, whether they did so simply by treading upon corrupted ground or actively trying to remove the poison. From the land, the water, a living body—treating the poison drained the mender in a manner unlike any other. Prolonged exposure to it eroded the body, and healing could only do so much for so long. Magic worked until it didn't, but thus far, no one had determined the magic-born poison's breaking point.

The only saving grace, double-edged as it was, lay in the strange fact that the poison was specifically tailored to seek the magic wellspring in Rhell. While the elective struggled to test their growing mixes in contaminated earth that went sterile once it passed into the Valley, the same reaction could be used in the favor of poisoned bodies as well as dirt. If caught in time, at any rate. Even the protections of the Valley had limits. Regardless, whatever fueled the poison, it cared only to destroy Rhell. For now, anyway.

But for Dae to need a refresher in the Valley after only a few months in Rhell? Eunny didn't like the sound of it. Even if Ezzyn was being overprotective—which was a distinct possibility considering how his middle brother, Garethe, was chronically ill merely from proximity to the poison, and Ezzyn wasn't taking any chances with Dae—that meant something.

They were shown into a room toward the back of the Healing Hut. Dae insisted that Eunny and Ezzyn be allowed in as well, despite the disapproving look from the aide escorting them. Ezzyn spoke quietly to the aide outside the door, showing them a letter he'd carried in his cloak pocket. The aide nodded once and departed, returning in what had to be record time with none other than the Chief Mender.

"I thought you said it wasn't serious," Eunny muttered, nudging Dae.

"It isn't, Miss Song," Chief Hakan said. "And we're going to ensure it stays that way."

A reflexive "Yes, sir," was out of her mouth before Eunny could stop it. She hid her disgruntlement by looking down, listening intently as the chief explained the multi-pronged healing he would work. She was several years past her student days, and even back then, she'd only had sporadic interactions with the Chief Mender. Apothecary-track didn't overlap much with someone of his standing, and especially not at the lower levels. That he'd somehow managed to remember her name should've been a crime.

Chief Hakan flicked clear the tails of his mender's jacket—ivory bordered in gold to denote his status—as he sat on a stool next to Dae. He took her hand between his own, her light brown skin pale in contrast to his golden brown. The chief took a measured breath in, held it for a beat as his magic surged, and exhaled at the same unhurried pace. Golden light flared between his palms, flowing into Dae as his head bent toward her. Dae, eyes closed, bowed her head as well.

Eunny crossed her arms, hands turning to fists as her magic woke in the presence of its own kind. It hummed in her veins like a sympathetic string, a quiet vibration in her blood. She ignored it, picturing herself as stone.

The healing session was over in the blink of an eye, Chief Hakan releasing Dae's hand and standing in one smooth motion. He went to the small counter at the back of the room and took down a cup and a few small jars. Using a set of silver menders' measuring spoons, he portioned out varying amounts of different powders from the jars along with a few sparks of his own magic for each addition.

Eunny's hands itched with the impulse to check his ratios, even though she knew the Chief Mender had dual Master levels for light magic, both in mending. Full track for body magic, and the research levels for herbalism. Had graduated with distinction, just to cement himself as the most overqualified Chief Mender in the history of Sylveren University, or some such nonsense. The man had probably forgotten more than she'd ever know about apothecary work.

Didn't stop her from craning her neck around to try and catch the labels on the jars.

"Professional interest, Miss Song?" the Chief Mender asked, his tone dryly amused.

"Nope, not anymore. Just stretching my neck." Wood-smoked sundew powder, some kind of mountain lettuce, and she couldn't see the farthest jar before he stored them away again. All good choices. Maybe not *exactly* what Eunny would've put together, but not objectionable. Not that she was thinking about going into apothecary work again. Stopping Ennis from turning their stomach to lead had been a one-time thing.

Chief Hakan brought the cup to Dae, offering it to her along with a small stirring rod. "Your magic will help the mending set, but I can ask one of the aides for a glass of water if you need." He glanced at Eunny before focusing on Dae. "I've strengthened the tissue in your lungs, but this should provide more fortification."

Dae accepted the cup with a murmur of thanks. She glanced at Ezzyn. "Could you open the window, please?"

He complied, revealing the gray skies and misty rain that had begun falling while they were inside. Dae made a beckoning motion, summoning a thin stream of moisture to form around her fingers before she directed it into the cup. A few stirs dissolved the powder, leaving behind a dark, greenish-brown liquid. Dae gave it a sniff and grimaced.

"Drink the whole thing, please." Chief Hakan motioned to Ezzyn. "I need to confer with Mr. Sor'vahl. Miss Song, I presume you remember standard protocol?"

Eunny flapped a hand at him. "Monitor her for a bit in case of adverse effects. I got it."

"I'm going to check in with Gaz, too, if I can find him," Ezzyn said. "I'll meet up with you—"

"At the greenhouse complex," Eunny interrupted. "I want to give Dae a tour later."

"Perfect. I need to make arrangements with the groundskeeper about soil samples, too."

Once Ezzyn and Chief Hakan had left and the door closed behind them, Dae's head whipped toward Eunny. "The greenhouse complex? Do tell."

"Says she who didn't mention a peep about this in her last letter," Eunny groused. She went to shut the window, resuming the privacy charm enchanted into each of the Healing Hut's rooms. "Since when does a prince of Rhell do dirt delivery?"

"It's for samples from the containment zones. Ez has been working with the glassblower guild on new shielding spells. Hopefully, we'll get the next batch to last several days. As for the letter"—a guilty smile flashed across Dae's face as she ducked her head in contrition—"I didn't want you to worry! Ez is overreacting."

Eunny dropped onto the Chief Mender's vacated stool. "Is he, though? Why're you getting personally treated by the chief if it's nothing serious?"

Dae choked down more of her medicinal brew. "It really isn't. Certainly not if it meant having to drink this, Great Wave drown me." She took another sip, meeting Eunny's skeptical gaze, and sighed. "The poison *is* getting stronger within containment zones. The wards are working, but it's like the poison is more... concentrated. The symptoms are unchanged, but it all hits faster now."

"Lovely," Eunny muttered. "Guess the secrecy makes sense."

"Tell me about you. The greenhouse? You didn't mention any of that in *your* last letter either, Lady Hypocrite." Dae pointed an accusing finger. "All you said was that the café needed some repairs."

"And that's the truth!"

"We rode past it on the way in, Eun. You never said it *collapsed*." Dae glowered at her. "What happened? Tell me everything and take my mind off the taste of this swill."

It was Eunny's turn to shrink inward. In stops and starts, she recounted the last day of Song's Scrap, of Ollas's injury and her own guilt. She cringed over the tale of her living situation, and softly admitted how she liked the Grove and assisting with Ollas's work.

"Are you thinking about bringing back some apothecary work?" Dae asked carefully, glancing back toward the cabinet where the Chief Mender had stored the jars.

"No. I don't know. Not really?" Eunny ran her fingers through her hair. "There's this side project Nev has been working on..."

Dae was quiet for a moment. "Oh? *Nev?*"

"Yea." Eunny made a face at her friend. "You've heard me—I've been calling him that since we were kids!"

Dae set the now-empty cup aside. "I don't recall that at all." She scooted forward on the examination chair. "Anyway, you were saying? You and Nev?"

"There are these plants—he grew them from seed stock the Sentinels found during the delegation mess. There's something about them. I think they might..." Eunny hesitated. She loved Dae, trusted her, but she'd been selling the story about having lost her magic for so long. Even to one of her best friends, she didn't know how to go about undoing years of lies. Easier to just add another to the pile.

"It'll be faster if I just show you." Eunny got to her feet. "It's been long enough. I'll vouch for your leaving."

They headed back down the road, cloak hoods pulled up against the light rain.

"Did you hear that my father formally stepped back from his director role at Helm Naval?" Dae asked. "Calya's already plotting her final takeover."

Dae's father had stubbornly held on to his title at the maritime trading company he'd built, Helm Naval Engineering, despite having moved on to a political position in Graelynd's minor council. A move—or lack of one—that had caused a growing amount of friction with his youngest daughter.

"Gods all help anyone who stands in her way," Eunny said.

"She's finalizing a new trade deal with Renstown. If you need anything from Central sent by a faster boat, just ask."

"Think she can cut out the Coalition?"

Dae laughed. "No harm in asking. I'm pretty sure Caly thrives on adversity."

Their talk turned to Eunny's attempts at playing grovetender. Dae wasn't surprised by the Restorers of the Alliance being involved with a class at Sylveren, and muttered darkly about the Coalition sponsorship. The timeframe elicited an eyeroll.

"One term! For a new hybrid? Even with accelerated growth boosters, that sounds more like politics and business than anything with a mind for research. *One term*," Dae muttered. "I'll bet the Coalition is behind pushing that kind of deadline. Ridiculous."

"You sound like N—Ollas." Eunny chuckled. "Though I think he secretly likes the challenge."

Dae gave her a sidelong glance. "You two seem to have gotten close."

"I'm his peon. Not for much longer, anyway. He doesn't really need my help anymore." Eunny's smile faltered, but she hitched it back into place when Dae continued to eye her.

"Do you want to stay?" Dae asked.

"Hard to make an excuse when he can haul his own dirt."

"I'm not talking about objectivity." Dae's tone became too innocent as she asked, "Does he want you to stay?"

Eunny stopped in the middle of the road. "Meaning?"

Dae tugged her back to walking. "You know, he always had a bit of a crush on you. Who wouldn't? I think half the town was in awe of you when you started coming up here to visit."

"Ollas doesn't— He's not— We're *friends*."

"And friendship is a beautiful thing. But I'll note that you don't seem entirely opposed to the idea."

"Still getting over the shock," Eunny grumped. "Aren't you nosy today?"

"As if you weren't ten times worse when I first started up with Ezzyn."

"It's not the same! I think the enthusiastically consensual hopping into bed made it clear you two were sharing the same brain. It was the eyeballs that were lacking."

Dae laughed, giving Eunny a playful shove. "You're terrible." She peered at Eunny, a wheedling note in her voice as she said, "Are you really telling me there's been nothing? No spark?"

"Not..." The memory of shirtless Ollas answering his door rose up in Eunny's head. Of nicely defined shoulders, light skin dusted with freckles. Gods, his freckles. How easy it was to make him flush. Then there was the pleased, possessive warmth that was always trying to spread through her belly. "Not that I can—"

"There is! You do have a spark."

Eunny remembered waking up and being covered by his blanket. She'd felt a pang of regret at waking up alone. She remembered all of it with a level of detail that meant something, and her willful ignorance was running out.

"Why do you look less than happy about this?" Dae asked. "I know he's not your usual type, but—"

"I don't have a *type*. And it's not a spark, it's just nerves and pent-up, you know"—Eunny gestured at nothing—"whatever."

Dae raised her eyebrows. "Sure, but if it was just some pent-up *whatever*, you could've hopped a boat to Renstown and had that friend of yours take care of it."

"Can't. He and the harbormaster's son finally committed." Eunny shrugged.

"Okay, fine, then you could've picked someone else. My point is, you didn't."

"Maybe my bag of flings is just empty."

"Sylvan is small, but it's not that small. And you've got the school, ships coming in regularly at the port. If you just needed to blow off steam, you could've. You didn't," Dae said. "Doesn't that tell you something?"

"I'll let you know," Eunny muttered.

"You do that."

They spent the next hour at the greenhouse, Eunny leading Dae on a tour of the elective's hybridization attempts and then back to the secret propagation attempt in Trunk. That Dae didn't feel anything beyond the ordinary with the plants, no pull or hint of arcane energy, left Eunny disquieted, though she tried not to show it. If the resonance wasn't attuned solely to magic, then what? Maybe she could drag in one of the Initiate One students with an affinity for light magic and see if they reacted.

"Are they for restoration work?" Dae asked.

"We're not sure," Eunny replied. Seeing Ezzyn walking up the path, deep in conversation with the greenhouse complex manager, she stuck the pot onto its shelf and ushered Dae back into the greenhouse's main room. "At this point, they're practically weeds."

Eunny glanced back at the secret pots. Her negligent slip-up with her magic hadn't changed the plant, but the intangible pull remained. It waited, a steady hum in the back of her mind, wanting more.

Before she could change her mind, she went back into the antechamber and snatched up the pot to send home with Dae. She and Ollas could always pot up a replacement—it wasn't like they were going to run out when they had an entire bed full of the things. Maybe the mages in Rhell would have more success. Or maybe Ollas was on to something and the plants were somehow attuned to him—and Eunny.

Only one way to find out.

Chapter Thirteen

BEING able to tromp around Sylveren's grounds without pain was the new height of luxury for Ollas. He wasn't fully recovered, but now his aches were the familiar kind of soreness. A dull pain that told him he hadn't worked those muscles in a while. It was the kind of feeling that said he was getting stronger. Which he hoped was true; hauling in a single sack of grow mix from Trunk to where the elective's work was housed in the Adept levels' main greenhouse, Sapling, had left him a sweaty mess. His curls were plastered to his temples, loose shirt clinging in places and probably adorned with stains to match.

A large clay pot sat on the ground near the greenhouse's long main counter. A philodendron had long since climbed out of its container and spread throughout the greenhouse, defying all attempts to prune and tame its growth. Ollas was pretty sure a variation of the plant had taken up residence throughout every building in the complex; not quite the same, but a guardian variety that had adapted to the different conditions. Its protection qualities had softened over the decades, maybe even centuries, of Sylveren's history, changing to reflect the latent magic collecting in the various greenhouses each iteration of the plant called home. Where the Magisters' greenhouse specimen was grace and power, with variegated, blade-shaped leaves the length of a forearm, the plant in the Adept levels' greenhouse was more robust. Dark green leaves the size and shape of dinner plates. A few splits, but nothing like the Magisters' plant. Not unlike the even bulkier cousin that lived in the Initiate greenhouse, the Sapling plant looked hearty, capable of withstanding the trials and tribulations of living in those years' buildings.

Ollas stuck his finger in the soil and reached for a trickle of his magic. Instead of a steady flow, his had always been more of a faucet with a slow leak—occasional drips that emerged at their own leisure. Tired as he was, it didn't surprise him when his magic's response was more of a fizzle. The lower leaves ruffled once, giving him the impression of mild annoyance. Not unlike a horse twitching to shoo a fly on its flank, not even worth the effort of a tail swish.

"Sorry, friend," he murmured, straightening up. His brief gleaning of the soil's contents didn't reveal anything aside from the standard potting mix. Given the age and level of entrenchment, Ollas guessed that the vine had other sources for nutrients throughout the greenhouse. The hearty stems thrummed with latent magic, some innate to the plant and some likely stored from so much exposure to young mages going about their work. He didn't recognize the signature, as it was, of the medley of spellwork within the leaves, but rather something inherent in the magic's structure. An old enchantment for roof integrity, perhaps? Or maybe a fire suppressant charm—the Initiate levels greenhouse had a full slate of fire, flood, and general explosion-proofing spells, along with general safety enchantments that were refreshed yearly. It seemed fitting to Ollas that the old protector vine would evolve to embody such defenses.

Giving the leaf a last admiring stroke with his finger, he noticed new growth at the base as the plant readied itself to flower. Going to the nearest counter, Ollas scrounged around until he found an old seed packet and stub of a pencil. He scribbled a note to himself on the back so he wouldn't forget to make changes to his lesson plan and incorporate it into his class. It was rare for these old philodendrons to bloom, between how long it took for them to grow to maturity and the decades-long cycle between blooming periods. Even then, the exact triggers that sent the plants into flowering were hard to predict with—

Ollas's hand jerked. He bolted upright, hissing in pain as his back protested. He ignored it, mind racing. It wasn't unheard of for flowering only to be brought on by the most discriminating convergence of conditions. In some cases, those triggers caused the plant to change in appearance. Like going from plain and grass-like to variegated and leafy?

Slowly, thoughts whirling together, Ollas left Sapling and made his way back toward Trunk. It was a wild theory, but everything about those delegation plants was a little unconventional. He'd submitted a request for the Sentinels' records on the delegation rescue and likely wouldn't hear back for at least a week, maybe longer. But he'd already started some propagation experiments, so what harm was there in trying a few more? He was keeping notes on the process per the school's standard guidelines, and Rai knew, vaguely, that Ollas was fussing with some old Trunk stock. So long as he covered expenses and kept the school informed, no one was likely to complain. Ollas doubted anyone was even paying attention, Trunk not being a hotbed for cutting edge research.

Once inside the storage greenhouse, Ollas's tired body forced him to rest. He settled onto a stool and stretched his bad leg out, wincing as his knee cracked. But at this point, any stiffness was temporary. He'd managed all his gardening duties, light though they were, all afternoon with minimal trouble. Which meant his days of needing Eunny's help were well and truly over. Which wasn't wholly bad; having to sit and watch had made him feel so inept.

But needing her? Just her. He couldn't call it *beginning*, not when he'd been ensorcelled for so long. But something had started to *change*. His wistful longing was turning into something more, felt like it had turned a corner, ascended a level. It felt like maybe, possibly, there was a chance for something real. She'd been willing to help out with his delegation plant experiment, even though she usually avoided anything to do with that awful time. Would she follow him down the path of this newest theory about the radical change in the plants? It was hard to imagine her slogging up from Sylvan, especially when he had no idea what exact conditions the plants needed to flower. The tedium of the elective's numerous trying-and-failing-to-start seeds had been bad enough.

But more than their greenhouse adventures, he liked having her in class, too. It was sort of like when someone audited a course. Considering that Eunny was a novice to grovetending and the elective was far above her level, she managed fine. Got along with the students, many of whom knew of her through her repair café or her aunt's teashop.

Ollas wanted her to stay. They were on the verge of...something. So many times, now, it had felt as if the affections he'd carried were about to culminate, to be revealed. And Eunny, she sensed it. In the carriage. The greenhouse. His godscursed kitchen table, his temporary *bed*, when he'd been so close to throwing caution to the wind and finally kissing her. Only it was his nerve that kept failing. Had him confessing feelings when he knew they couldn't be heard. He might as well not have said anything at all.

With a groan that was only partly due to his aching joints,

Ollas grabbed a trowel and went out to the overgrown section behind Trunk to gather more fodder for his propagation experiments. He knelt, sinking his fingers into the loosened earth. Taking a deep breath, Ollas mentally reached for any remnants of his magic. A few drops came to him, wicking into the soil much easier than he'd expected. But then the magic was gone, and the plants didn't have even the slightest aura of the arcane about them.

Unperturbed, he dug up another clump and levered himself back up to his feet in time to see Eunny coming toward him.

"Look at you, no cane or anything. Guess I'm out of a job," she teased.

"Yeah, I..." Ollas paused, glancing at her as he murmured, "Can we not, just for—just for a little bit, can we not talk about you..."

"Me?" Eunny said, drawing out the word. "Me, what, exactly?"

"Leaving."

"Oh. Sure." Faint spots of color appeared on her cheeks. "Sorry, I, uh—" She blinked, a frazzled note in her voice. "I forgot to tell you that I sent Dae home with one of your secret plants."

"Ours now, or are you backing out on me?" Ollas joked. "I have a theory on why they're changing." He quickly explained his idea about the plants changing for a bloom cycle as they went back into Trunk.

"Okay," Eunny said slowly, helping him gather an assortment of propagation supplies. "So, you think these are one of those special 'blooms once a century' kind of things?"

"Not a century, but something like that." Ollas dragged out the old ledger with its one sparse entry pertaining to the seeds-now-turned-plants. Finger skimming across his faded scrawl, he tapped one spot. "Six years ago, we were having an unseasonable amount of rain."

Eunny didn't look convinced. "It rains all the time here. We're having a lot now, but is that really all it takes?"

"Well... No, probably not in this case," Ollas admitted. "We're missing something else, but it's a start!"

Ollas poured imbued mineral additive into a tray, adding a healthy scoop of worm castings before wetting the lot with enriched water and giving it all a rough mix with his hand. He picked up a glass stirring rod with an icy blue core. "If you were a grovetender or I was a better one, we could use magic to augment the mix in the pots I've already got started. It's not hard, but it works best with consistency, and my magic isn't that. Easier to just do it the mundane way."

He demonstrated, showing her how to move the rod throughout the tray he'd assembled, dispersing the line of blue from within the glass. It came out like a gel, wanting to clump rather than spread. Ollas showed her how he kept a finger in the soil at all times, feeling the cold tingle of the ice magic.

Then he offered the stirring rod to her. Eunny took it, hesitating with the glass still held aloft. "Me? What if I screw it up?"

"That's grovetending," he replied with a smile. He cleared his throat, head ducking down as he mumbled, "I was, uh, hoping you'd want to be involved."

Eunny gave him a curious look, her lips quirking in a playfully suspicious moue as she set the tip of the rod into the mix. But she did it.

Ollas picked up a fresh rod. "Too much and it clumps or goes blocky. Too little and it won't feel even." He nudged a sodden blob near the edge of the tray with his stirring rod. "Go until the rod is clear and the mix feels cool but kind of fluffy."

Eunny speared a clump. "Why didn't we do this with the other ones?"

"This is a lot of imbued amendment to throw at it. Most seedlings would die, but these plants are... strange. It's like they absorb magic."

Eunny didn't comment. He watched her from the corner of his eye, trying not to be too obvious. She frowned down at her mix, brow furrowing in concentration. She held the rod in a death pinch, fingertips going white from the pressure.

"Little softer. Treat it like a pen," Ollas said. "It won't jump away from you."

She complied, somewhat, letting blood flow back into her fingers, though her motion was still rigid. Her other hand, the one monitoring the mix, was another story. She traced through the material with her index finger, the rest curled loosely against her palm. On occasion, she would let one dangle, like dipping her toes into water, as she followed the tray's rim. She moved from the wrist, graceful, minute turns for changes of angle.

"Am I doing it wrong?" Eunny asked, raising her brows at him. "You're staring, Professor."

Heat surged through his groin. Which he really, *really* didn't need right now, not when there was a good chance that her very presence would pique his cock's interest even more. He didn't have the handy escape of going to check on other students. And if Eunny noticed... Gods. He'd have to leave the country. If he didn't drop dead from embarrassment first.

"I'm admiring." He gestured toward the tray. "Your technique."

Eunny snorted, giving the mix a vigorous stir.

Ollas spun around and pretended to rummage through the pots on the opposite counter. "How does the mix feel now?"

"Cold. Kind of dry, but not really, because I can see how it took up the water."

Ollas nodded as she talked, nudging his troublesome cock

up and trapping it behind the confines of his belt. Taking advantage of the trailing vines hanging from the ceiling, his movements were decently hidden.

"I guess it's fluffy." Eunny held up her now-clear stirring rod. "Does this mean it worked?"

Ollas resumed his place next to her and tested the mix, nodding with approval. "It's prepared correctly. We should have an idea of whether or not it's doing anything in a day or so."

He made a shallow impression for the new plant, gently pressing the roots down into the mix before putting a thin layer of it over the top.

"Great. Waiting. My favorite." Eunny carried the tray into the rear antechamber and placed it next to its sibling plants on the lower shelf. When she straightened, she nudged Ollas's arm. "We should probably talk about how you don't need my help anymore."

The quiet statement was enough to make his cock droop. It softened, falling free from his waistband, limp and sad as he felt.

"Thanks for this. Letting me help. I know I kind of bullied you into it." A sheepish grin lit her face. "But it's been fun, being back here. Doing the school thing again. I'd forgotten what it feels like."

"To be a student?"

Eunny wasn't looking at him, her gaze drifting around the greenhouse. Taking it all in as if for the last time. "To be a part of all this," she murmured. "I'll miss it."

"But you already are. What about the work you've done for the school?" Ollas protested.

Her gaze was fixed on the window, but her focus was somewhere else. Inside. Lingering over that which he couldn't see. "Maybe I was once, but I'm not a part of this place anymore. I left and never looked back." She tilted her head toward him, a sad smile on her face. "Until you. I don't know what to think about that. It feels like it should be wrong, but..."

He didn't understand. Was on the cusp of saying as much, but Eunny already seemed to know.

She sighed. "It's never felt... right, coming back. To the town, to the school, the Valley. Take your pick. Not because I'm uncomfortable with magic. I'm *mad*. Because it fucking failed me. It failed when I needed it most, and I don't know why. It failed in the worst way possible. I'm supposed to heal people, and instead my magic ruined you."

"You didn't," Ollas murmured. He ached to say more, to take her guilt and anger and tear it into shreds, but she stopped him with a weary shake of her head.

She picked a dead leaf from the length of vine nearest to her and began tearing it into pieces. "I've been able to call light since before I could walk. Could imbue Auntie Yerina's cold remedy blends before I could see over the counter. I don't know what magic is like for you, but I've known mine forever. It was like breathing. So for it to go so badly, for it to have been so natural and then become unknown... I don't know how to come back from that. I'm trained, Nev, I did all my schooling. I learned what the consequences are supposed to be of pushing beyond your limits, same as everyone else. Magic fails sometimes, but then it should've failed *me*. Should've hurt *me*, not you. But it didn't."

His hand twitched toward her, hesitating in midair. He wanted to touch her, hold her, absorb any of her sorrow that he could if it meant that she would carry less of it.

When she didn't move away, he placed his hand over hers.

She gave him a grim smile. "I don't remember much of that day. That part is true, but it's by choice. When I think about it, when I remember... I can't just remember it. I have to live it, and that sucks."

He squeezed her hand.

"It was the only time my magic's ever gotten away from me." Eunny laughed once, the sound devoid of any mirth. "Everyone harps on me to get my magic back, because how could you want to go from magic to mundane if given the choice? Gods, it was so easy." Her fingers wrapped tightly around his. "The life I used to have? Apothecary work. I don't want—" Her head jerked sharply. "It's not for me anymore."

For a while, neither spoke. Ollas looked down at their entwined hands. At hers, still so beautiful in his eyes. But her hands were not without pain. Not so innocent, despite appearances. He wouldn't claim to understand all the horror she'd felt, but Ollas couldn't call himself a stranger to such feelings, either. If only.

"I'd never seen the Sentinels kill before that day," Ollas said, his voice low even in the quiet emptiness of the greenhouse. "We'd gotten into some scrapes, fights with poachers, rogue mages trying to sneak across the border, that sort of thing. Had to cull an entire herd of elk over by the Earthen Run one winter when disease broke out. We train more to subdue, bring them in for the Order's magistrate to sort it out. I'd never struck at someone and meant for them to stay down."

Eunny mulled over his words, her gaze back to some point far beyond the window.

"Six years later and I'm still"—he shrugged—"conflicted."

"And now you can't get real closure. I took that from you," she murmured. "I'm so—"

Ollas chuckled softly. "I don't need to be swinging a sword around to feel my feelings. Eunny, it wasn't your fault."

"Having a positive attitude about me turning you into a safety liability doesn't make it not my fault."

Hesitantly, Ollas reached for her, fingers soft against her cheek as he coaxed her to face him. "I can still do routine forestry work. I *like* that stuff. And now with teaching full time again…" He slowly lowered his hand. "It all works—"

Eunny caught his hand, held on as she asked in a fierce, low voice, "And you're happy with that?"

"Yes. The Sentinels gave me so much, especially when I was young and just this gangly weed, too shy to make friends." Ollas let himself lean ever so slightly into her touch. "But I was never a *real* ranger. I'm a gardener. This way, I get to do both. I just wish things could've been easier for you."

"You're *really* okay with—with this? With everything?" Eunny clasped his cheeks between her hands.

Ollas tried to nod.

"*Really?*"

He laughed, earning the beginning of a smile from her in return. "Yes, really."

Eunny peered at him with exaggerated scrutiny, then slowly released his face. Ollas thought he felt a slight quaver run through her fingers, but she smirked at him, patting his chest before turning back to the counter. "Well, that settles that. Gods, we got dreary for a moment, didn't we?" She gestured at the rest of the greenhouse, then gave him a pointed look. "Still doesn't change that you're healed enough to not need me around anymore."

"There's a place for you here, if you want it," he said. "There's plenty of work to be done still, even if I don't strictly *need* the physical help. I'm not going to turn it away."

"You do remember that I'm not a grovetender, right? I've been here for a month, and I'm not sure I've actually grown anything myself. At all."

"I think I can convince Rai." In a hesitant voice, he added,

"We're ready to start evaluating the healing properties in the plants."

"Apothecary work, eh?" Eunny sounded tired, but not outright against it.

"Assessments. You could do it using the mundane approach. We need to test use cases for anyone doing restorative work, anyway. No magic required."

"Really don't want to get rid of me, eh?"

"No," Ollas said, voice serious despite her joking manner. "I-I want you to stay."

Eunny blinked at him. "I—" Her mouth quirked up. "Well, if you're going to say it like that, then I accept. Or rather, I'm fine with staying until I'm told to go."

"Really?"

"I mean, we're talking about research that directly affects Dae." She shrugged. "And you're a good teacher, Nev. You make it... easier, to be here. Be around magic."

"I'm glad." Ollas hesitated, then said softly, "Thanks, for telling me about all of it."

"Feels weird. It's usually easier to pretend."

"Why did you stop?"

She glanced sidelong at him. "I guess because I didn't want to like you earlier."

Ollas was silent for a few long, full seconds as her words rang through his ears. Slowly, he swung around to face her. "Does that mean you do now?"

"I..." Eunny tried to sound nonchalant, but a spot of pink was back on her cheeks.

They both startled as the outer door to the greenhouse banged open. Gransen bustled in. "Olly? You in here?"

"I'll—" Eunny glanced down. In their surprise at being interrupted, she'd bumped against Ollas, her arm brushing his thigh.

Heat rose in his face. And other places. Ollas coughed nervously, angling his torso away, flush intensifying when Eunny tried, and failed, to smother a cackle.

"I take it back," she murmured, grabbing an armload of the planting supplies they'd used. "Guess I can make one thing grow."

If there was a time in his life where Ollas had ever been more mortified yet painfully aroused at the same time, he couldn't recall.

Eunny *winked* at him, then in a louder voice, she called, "What do you want, gremlin?"

Ollas heaved an inward sigh once her back was to him and she'd gone to intercept Gransen. In a maneuver that was becoming far too practiced, he flipped his hardened dick back up beneath his waistband. And he tried, with little success, not to think about Eunny's wicked delight in making him grow.

Chapter Fourteen

EUNNY DUCKED out of her room, quieting her step as she went through the empty common area to the door. Ollas was back to sleeping in his own bed, the living area returned to a shared communal space. Papers were strewn across the table, a mix of Gransen's studies, Ollas's midterm prep, and various correspondence related to the elective. Eunny retrieved a piece that had fallen on the floor, lips twitching into a smile when she saw Ollas's blocky handwriting.

A ramp-up in work hadn't spared them much in the way of privacy since their talk in the greenhouse. Days turned into a week, and though he still flushed at her jokes, and laughter and conversation flowed easily between them, there was something else in the air now, too. Something charged. Glances that lingered a beat too long to be nothing. And, if she was honest with herself, those looks weren't happening only one way.

Ollas had been true to his word, getting her added on as some sort of vaguely official consultant for the elective. She didn't know how he'd sold it to Rai and didn't ask. Ollas hadn't said anything about their almost...whatever it was that had happened between them. That crystalline moment when she'd let her mouth run off and spill her angry heart. Spilled some feelings, too. Tested the air to see if the spark Dae kept asking about really existed.

And, oh, did it ever. The feel of Ollas's hand on hers. His quiet, earnest words. The way he looked at her. Not to mention his other bodily reactions. It was unsettling, how she craved more. Which was unlike her. She didn't mean to brag or anything, but whenever she'd deigned to "hop a boat to Renstown," as Dae had put it, Eunny didn't lack for choice. Her singledom of the last several years was of her own volition, a mix of busyness and apathy.

That had been her outlook since she'd settled in the Valley. And yet, Eunny was pretty damn sure that if Gransen hadn't barged in on them, she'd have learned if that spark she felt with Ollas had a taste.

Which was exciting *and* a problem. She felt...safe, around him. No, not safe. Safety implied fear, and she wasn't afraid of her traitorous magic. More like incandescent with rage. But, just with his presence, Ollas softened those emotions, too. She felt *comfortable* with him. Calmer. Enough to consider dabbling a bit more. Which was folly. Magic was dead to her, apothecary work just a thing of her past. Eunny was here to assuage her guilt, not to test out her magic. Not to make herself feel at home. Freckles and a few soft touches didn't undo six years of feeling destroyed.

But damn did being around Ollas nearly do it. As evidenced by her still being here. Giving commentary on the elective's medicinal trials. Fending off Ennis and their pestering about how to steep the ultimate brain elixir or whatever else they were trying on any particular day. Eunny even had a water propagation setup in her windowsill for a few pieces of the delegation plants. None of it required her magic, but such distinction felt more and more like a technicality. She was supposed to have left this aspect of her life behind. These allowances she kept making, letting herself feel comfortable, none of it could last. Eunny knew it yet didn't feel bothered by it. She happily pushed those whispers of concern aside.

Taking a detour so she could pass through the Heartwood, Eunny snagged a biscuit from a plate Soph had left out to share. She gave it a tentative sniff—no lavender this time, but a delicious bite of mint. Lingering by the table, she eavesdropped as a group of Initiate Ones engaged in vigorous debate over how to improve a humane mouse trap for the Heartwood's resident terrors.

"It ruined my wheat berries. I say we just get a trap from town."

"We're *Sylveren grovetenders*! We can build better than—"

"I told you not to use Soph's nut butter."

"Hey! It's fresh-churned, no preserva—"

"It's a *mouse*. It wants the cheap shit they eat in Central."

Covering a smile behind her pilfered biscuit, Eunny turned to the door in time to see Zhenya walking by, arms full with two large packages.

"Mail run?" Eunny asked, intercepting her friend and relieving her of one of the parcels.

Zhenya nodded, murmuring her thanks as she said, "Copy of my thesis on interdisciplinary ink applications for pictorial enchantments."

"Explains why this feels like a ton of books." Eunny hefted her package. "With all your studying, how are you not at Master level yet?"

Zhenya laughed, nudging the Heartwood's outer door open for them. "I'd have to get through Magister's first."

"What's the hold up?"

"I get distracted." Zhenya indicated the package in her hands. "Samples from the red dye plants I was working on for

Adept Two. These are for a friend in southern Graelynd working on improving archival colors. Doesn't count for Magister One since it's all old research."

Eunny shook her head. Zhenya could earn all three Magister levels if she'd set her mind to it. The little inkmaker loved the university, that much was plain, but for whatever reason, she didn't strive for a higher rank or profession. She was content to stay an Adept Two and senior assistant for Professor Rai. Eunny coveted such happiness. Divested as she was from her mother's meddling, she still hadn't completely banished the nagging sense of obligation to do more, always.

They split up at the mailroom's counter, Zhenya to post her packages and Eunny to check the box she'd been sharing with Ollas and Gransen during her stay. It was too soon for Dae to have written, but Yerina sent up relevant correspondence whenever any came in.

Several envelopes stuffed the small box. Most were for Gransen and Ollas, with only a few for Eunny. The short, terse note from her mother nagging for an update was easily tossed out, but a flare of guilt licked at her when she found an envelope with her aunt's flowy handwriting. She'd been lax in getting back into town of late. It had been weeks now since Bioon's second surprise visit, and Eunny had only seen her aunt for a handful of minutes the few times she'd been by the Mighty Leaf.

Her guilt intensified when she saw that Yerina's letter, aside from some notes on early planning for that year's Winterfest event at the teashop, also included estimates for the café's repairs from several craftspeople in Sylvan. Eunny flipped through the papers, noting price quotes and estimates for the time to start and complete different stages of work. She would have to decide who to hire and for what, soon, before schedules were booked up and the café suffered even more damage as it moldered away in its ruptured state.

Folding the papers back into the envelope, Eunny saw she had one last piece of mail. A half slip of paper bearing the bronze seal of Sylvan's administration department and the letterhead of the housing office. A small apartment over in Belle Complex was finally available if she still wanted it.

Did she? It would mean losing the Grove, her easy living situation, one short hallway separating her from Ollas and Gransen. No more guarantees of seeing them every day.

No interruptions from errant roommates.

"What's that?" Zhenya asked as she came over.

Eunny showed her the paper. Zhenya made a sound of approval. "Belle would be nice. Not too far from the greenhouses, and next door to the library."

Eunny snorted. "Now if only they could have books in an arboretum, we'd never see you again."

"I have some ideas for one," Zhenya said. "Small scale, but I might be able to get the humidity levels to work."

"I've no doubt." Eunny noticed the handful of envelopes Zhenya had retrieved from her own box. "Good mail day for you."

"Reports from some colleagues in Den'olm. We're almost ready to send them samples from the elective."

The border town in northeastern Rhell was one of the kingdom's main lines of defense against the poison due to its placement along a ley line. Containing the blight there took an immense amount of resources, and that was before calculating the extra time it took with the mages having to take trips to the Valley to purge the contamination from their bodies.

"Yea, Ollas is all aflutter about that," Eunny said. "He's going to end up back at the Healing Hut if he doesn't take a break."

The first trial had progressed to the point of flowering, the starter and transplant mixes now so finely tuned that if a batch suffered, the students could get a new flat planted and grown to size in a couple of days. The blooms produced were on the pale side, balanced atop delicate stems that defied gravity through what Eunny could only presume was grovetender sorcery. A cross-country trip seemed ambitious.

"We'll give them another run or two for improvements, but we can't accurately simulate the way the poison is reacting in containment," Zhenya said. "Even with the new shipments, the newer soil's just not lasting long enough down here to test those parameters."

Dae had confessed that Ezzyn was at loggerheads with his eldest brother, King Jeron, over whether or not to pause the containment efforts to ensure a supply of material for continuing research, or stay the course in deploying wards to curtail the spread. Eunny didn't envy them the conflict, for it seemed like choosing between evils. She knew Ezzyn could be zealous in his quest to find a cure for Rhell, but perhaps having the love of his life fall ill would tilt him toward his brother's approach.

"If we can get the seedlings to survive transplanting in Rhell, they'll have a shot at adapting," Zhenya continued. "We need a bit of luck. The Restorers are getting spooked about people getting sick faster."

Eunny muttered a few unkind words about investors safe in their beds in Graelynd, but her mind was stuck on something else. The plants and needing to grow in the place of corruption —something about it stuck in her head, but she couldn't quite parse out why. Dae and the visit at the Healing Hut kept flickering at the back of her mind.

"Oh! Before I forget, can you pass this on to Ollas?" Zhenya handed her another envelope. "He mentioned you're doing some research on the plants growing outside Trunk."

"Trying to, anyway. Whether that's wise or not." Eunny shrugged, quickly changing the subject. "Where are you headed now?"

Zhenya glanced at the wall clock by the door. "Slowly make my way back to the office and work on the Professor's report for Den'olm. You?"

"Get my stuff packed." Eunny paused. "Why 'slowly' going to the office?"

Zhenya hid a smile. "Professor Rai had an...appointment, this afternoon."

Eunny's head snapped up. "Are you telling me that *Saren Rai* and Garethe Sor'vahl are currently, as we speak, fu—"

Zhenya made hissing, shushing sounds and motions, her face going scarlet. Eunny laughed—maybe cackled—in response. That the two professors were romantically involved was perhaps the worst-kept secret on campus, but she never would've thought Rai, so proper and dignified, dare she say even a touch fussy, would be inclined toward anything remotely naughty. Garethe Sor'vahl, on the other hand...

The fragmented thoughts that had been floating around in Eunny's head for days began to click into place. Garethe Sor'-vahl, the middle brother, mundane but heavily invested in environmental restoration and how magic could be utilized to save his homeland. He also suffered from chronic illness caused by the poison, despite long periods of time away from any corrupted areas. Ezzyn had rushed Dae to the Valley for healing, for fear that her sickness might become anything like what plagued Garethe. While an entire summer spent in the Valley had improved Garethe's condition, he was far from cured.

There was a connection: illness and poison and the design of the remedy Dae had imbibed in the Healing Hut. She just couldn't figure out the order for it to make sense. Maybe a visit with Garethe was in order.

She glanced at Zhenya, who looked torn between being mortified and fighting giggles. Garethe could wait until tomorrow. Eunny had to pack for her relocation to Belle. Fortunate that she didn't have much stuff to move.

Leaving Zhenya to her slow return to the faculty branch, Eunny confirmed her new lodging with the housing office, then hurried back to the Grove.

Finding spare crates for the assortment of things she'd acquired took longer than the packing up. Gransen had absconded with the hand cart she'd originally brought. By the time Eunny found it and piled her stuff in the common room in a manner she was reasonably sure wouldn't topple over, Ollas had returned from his last office hours.

"Zhen has something for you," she said, pointing to where she'd left the envelopes from her mail run.

Ollas perked up, hurrying over to break the wax seal. His eyes flew across the page, then up to her. "It's about the delegation plants."

"She got the Sentinels' records?"

"No, they're still looking, too, but Zhen is friends with one of the archive clerks and got us some notes." Ollas handed her a slip of paper.

"What am I looking at?" Eunny asked. There was a botanical drawing and a block of text with lots of grovetender jargon and plant parts that she didn't understand.

"I'm positive that our plants are getting ready to bloom. Still not sure what they are, but they fit a lot of the criteria for rare bloom cycles," Ollas said. "Weather conditions. Remember the note about all the rain? We're having that again now. There must be a time element, too, since nothing induced them to change until now. And, I think it's us. Source magic."

Eunny frowned, setting the letter back onto the table. "Nev, but I don't... I've never put magic into those plants."

But that wasn't entirely true. The night she'd fallen into the garden flashed through her mind. The plants had still been those grassy mounds back then. Some of her magic had escaped. A small amount. Surely not enough to set off this rare bloom event Ollas was on about. And the few drops she'd accidentally summoned over the little cutting he was trying to grow? That was nothing. It couldn't be.

Ollas was oblivious to her rampaging thoughts. He began to pace, emphasizing his words with swipes of his hand. "I had them on me during the rescue. I'd been digging through the cache, and when the fighting broke out, I just stuck them in my pocket and ran out to help. When your magic went... when all that happened, what if the seeds absorbed it? We've seen how the plants seem to just take up magic. What if they're storing it and it's part of what gets them to flower?"

Eunny lowered herself into a chair at the kitchen table. It was possible, she supposed. Even if she was a terrible gardener and preferred to buy her herbalism wares already harvested, the practice of imbuing seed stock was common for the varieties with which it worked.

"Okay, maybe, *maybe,* I can believe some of that," she said. "But why now?"

"I think it's us," Ollas repeated. "Our magic. An imprinting spell—they're used sometimes to control supply. Seeds that'll only grow for specific magic-users. Or, in this case, flower. You've felt it, too, haven't you? The pull they have. It's been building for weeks. Months."

Eunny's mouth opened, her lips forming a denial. But... that restlessness, the unnamed certainty she'd been feeling. *I think it's us.* The eye twitches that had been plaguing her since summer.

Since Ollas had returned to Sylvan to resume teaching. And the plants had only changed once she'd come back to the school. Since she'd fallen in the garden bed, fed them more magic that had, in turn, caused them to change.

Ollas stopped in front of her, eyes alight. "Now we have direction. *Light magic.* We can tailor the amendments and treatments for that, see if we can get them to bloom."

"I don't have any magic to give," Eunny said weakly.

Ollas shrugged. "Even on my best of days, I don't have much." He shook his head, optimism rolling off him in joyous waves. "We can bring the ingredients in from other sources. I'll have to research imprinting spells more, but... will you try this with me?"

Seeing him so excited, it was hard not to feel the same. It filled her with a warmth, affection, and a swell of pleasure to be so wanted. A smile tugged at her lips.

She tapped her fingers together as she thought aloud. "Eyllic seeds. Fired up with my old magic." She glanced up at him. "We thinking healing properties?"

Ollas grinned. "Let's find out."

"Deal."

Ollas's laugh faded as he looked around, slowly comprehending the additional crates on the floor. "You're leaving?" he said, eyes sweeping over her bags, dismay in his voice.

"They finally had a place open up in Belle. I appreciated the room"—she waved back to the adjoining door—"truly, but I'd be lying if I said I didn't want something full-size."

Ollas cracked a smile. "Can't blame you for that." He sighed, the sound wistful as he stuck his hands in his pockets and shrugged. "I'll miss you."

"Not going far. I got promoted, remember? From packhorse to...whatever I am now. Lapsed apothecary who won't leave. *And* now, your secret lab partner."

"Won't be the same."

"True. I can think of a few differences." Eunny slowly

walked over until she stood in front of him. "I've been doing a lot of thinking about this. Because I still owe you an answer, don't I?"

The knob at his throat twitched with his swallow. "Y-Yes?"

His hazel eyes were mostly dilated now, pupils so large and dark that Eunny could easily see her grin in the reflection. His mouth dropped slightly open, leaving him looking equal parts awestruck and eager. This close, she could see that his freckles dusted more than his nose, the spots a mix of tiny specks and larger dots. She wondered if they existed elsewhere, if they were scattered across his body like stars. She wanted to trace each constellation, see what reactions her touch could bring. See if she could make him spark.

"Do you remember what I said back in the greenhouse?" She put her hand flat against his chest and smiled to feel how his muscles shivered in response.

"You said—" Ollas had to clear his throat. "You said something about making things, er, grow."

Eunny laughed. "Before that, Nev."

"That you didn't want to like me? Before."

"That part. I did say that," she agreed, nodding. Her fingers slid up to touch his neck. "What else?"

Ollas held himself still. Taut. "And I asked if that meant you do now."

"Yes, and then we were so rudely interrupted." She let her fingertips skim the stubble along his jaw. "But I think I've got my answer. Because you know the nice thing about me having my own place?"

Ollas held his breath. Eunny lifted her chin until she was inches from his mouth. "I do like you, Nev, and in Belle, we'll never get interrupted."

She meant to kiss him. Lightly. A flirty peck to test the waters, let him know she was game if he was. She loved this moment, the tension as those last pieces of the unknown between them fell away. The potential of everything they could be, before reality set a frame of reference. Of comparison. Drawing out the mystery, the possibility, she savored it.

She wasn't expecting shy, respectful, gentlemanly Ollas to grab her face and crash his mouth into hers. Wasn't expecting him to be so hungry, wasn't expecting the way his tongue invaded. There was nothing timid about the way Ollas cupped her chin and angled her mouth to his liking. The growl that came from him when she stroked his tongue with her own could be described with a variety of words, but none of them would be *shy*. He crushed Eunny to him, his hand spanning the small of her back.

She let her hands rove over his shoulders, his torso, reveling in the strength she found. Big hands. Thick fingers. A firm grip. Her nipples tightened at the thought of what this aggressive side of Ollas might do to her if given any encouragement.

She wasn't the only one having parts go firm. When he shifted and drew her against him, she pressed into his thigh and felt the bulge there. The prodding through the constraint of his trousers, in much more detail than the brief touch she'd had before.

Eunny choked. "Oh, shit, Nev." She looked down, saw the outline along the inside of his leg. "You're an animal."

Ollas froze. Being so close, she *felt* the moment realization caught up with him.

He sprang back. "Oh, oh, gods all... Fuck, Eunny, I'm so sorry."

She stared at him, then couldn't stop the cackle that broke free. She could've fried an egg on his face, it was so red.

"No, Nev, this is—" She could barely keep from devolving into snort-laughs. "Better I know now. Forewarned and forearmed and all of that, right? Oh, Goddess, I am going to need to be prepared!"

Ollas hid his face in his hands. "Earthen, please kill me."

"No, not before I get a chance to sample the—"

"What is all this ruckus? You know, you can hear it all the —" Gransen stopped in the doorway. He looked at Eunny, then looked at Ollas, who was still covering his face. Then, failing at any sense of self-control, Gransen looked down. "Should I go?"

Eunny smothered another laugh. "No, no, I'm on my way out." She went to the handcart and rummaged through her bag on top for the envelope from Yerina. She slapped it against Gransen's chest as she hauled the cart toward the door. "Look through these and help me with a shortlist for the café. We need a budget."

Gransen gasped, eyes going wide.

Eunny paused in the doorway, glancing back at Ollas, who was fiddling with his pockets. "I'll see you later?" She tilted her head toward him, feeling her smile all the way to the corners of her eyes.

As she trundled down the hall, she heard a light clap of hands on cheeks, followed by Gransen's solemn voice. "Boy, you are going to get fornicated."

Chapter Fifteen

It wasn't all in his head. Eunny was interested, too. Ollas hadn't imagined it. The way she'd touched him. Caressed his face. Ollas was mostly sure she'd been flirting, not that he was ever a good judge of such things. But he'd swear by every god in the Empyrean Court that she'd been about to kiss him before he'd attacked her with his face. Not that he was good at judging those likelihoods, either. And then he'd almost fucked it all up, giving in to his baser desires like the godsdamned animal she'd proclaimed him to be.

Though, Eunny hadn't *exactly* seemed to mind. Ollas felt a certain kind of satisfaction knowing that he'd surprised her. Pleasantly so.

I am going to need to be prepared.

It had taken every scrap of strength he possessed not to blow his load right then and there.

The interest was mutual, no doubt there. But since she'd left and Ollas had had a moment for his blood to flow somewhere besides straight to his dick, doubt had set in. Eunny said *later*, but how long was that? Was it too presumptuous to go by that same night? Gransen said no, but Gransen also possessed no shame. Plus, Eunny was moving. Unpacking. Maybe she'd want some time to get settled.

Ollas had been fantasizing about this day for years, but he had the sneaking suspicion that Eunny's interest was much more recent. Hard to tell. Her outgoingness, the jokes, her wickedly arousing teasing, they'd had that kind of lighthearted friendship for years. But that was just who Eunny was—it had never become anything more, and Ollas had been such a chickenshit he'd never had the nerve to make a move. He'd been content with being friends, his pining kept quietly under wraps. Until now. If he ruined everything, if she left Sylveren because of him, what then?

Ollas made the grave error of voicing some of those fears aloud, prompting Gransen to forcibly eject him from their room with a meaningful, "A gentleman is always prepared."

Which Ollas was not, and a trip to the university's student-run mercantile had given him a whole host of new things to agonize over.

What kind of contraceptive potion to acquire? One made by a Magister level, to be sure, but flavor? They'd been living together—sort of—for over a month now, but Ollas promptly forgot everything about what Eunny seemed to like. The variety pack seemed a safe choice, but multiple potions, gods, as if showing up the same day wasn't forward enough. Arriving at her door looking like he was set for a *very* good time... Ollas wouldn't blame her if she slammed it in his face instead.

He'd started to put the quartet of slim bottles back on the shelf, but then the thought of how Eunny had laughed flickered through his head. Her wicked glee at his... enthusiasm. He wanted it again. Wanted to be the one who brought her such delight, always.

The thought of tasting honey or three different types of fruit and berries on her lips was a motivator, too. The kind that had him pulling the fronts of his cloak close so he didn't risk embarrassment in the student store.

It had only been a couple of hours since Eunny had left. Far too soon to make an appearance. Ollas returned to the Grove, but when he went to open his door, it hardly budged.

"What the—?" Ollas tried again. A sliver of light appeared as the door opened a crack, thudding against something solid. "Granse? What happened to—"

"Olly, beloved, please," Gransen's voice floated through the door. "Do not be a *fool.*"

Muttering under his breath, Ollas put his shoulder against the wood and pushed. He didn't gain much, just enough to see that Gransen had piled a bunch of their shit on the other side, before the gremlin shoved back and the door closed once more.

"Gransen!"

Stranded out in the corridor, Ollas felt a prickle of concern as a few of the other residents went by. The bottle-filled sack hanging from his arm clinked in the tell-tale way that such glass bottles did, drawing more than one glance his way as Ollas tried to force the door in a nonchalant manner.

"Everything all right, Nevin?" his next-door neighbor asked.

"Yea, it's great, everything's great. Just Granse's idea of a joke, you know how—"

"If your dick's not wet, you're not—"

Godsdamn motherfucking... "I'm going, you bastard," Ollas hissed.

Pinching the bridge of his nose between his fingers, he ducked out, stuffing the bag into his cloak pocket.

The walk to Belle Complex had never felt so long in Ollas's life. If he'd been in a more rational state of mind, he'd recognize that it only took around fifteen minutes because it took all his self-control not to run the distance. Or turn around and slink back home, except that Gransen had removed that as an option.

Anticipation had him by the throat. By turns, it morphed between excitement and waves of insecurity. Ollas knew he made an amusing sight, shifting between an assured, steady pace and staggering nearly to a halt as indecision turned his boots to lead.

He forced himself on until, somehow, he was standing outside Eunny's door. A stroke of luck, his finding it in the first place, since he'd only realized once arriving at Belle that she hadn't given him a unit number. But he'd seen the assortment of teapots and cups she loved arranged on a windowsill, their mishmash of colors bright against the drawn curtains.

Taking a deep, steadying breath that did nothing for his nerves, Ollas knocked on the door.

The shuffling of feet and muted thump of a crate and flesh and the wall all making contact drifted through the wood to reach Ollas's ears. As did the grumbled curse that followed. He was covering a smile behind his hand when Eunny appeared in the doorway, standing on one leg as she rubbed her foot.

Her wince vanished at the sight of him, replaced by a mischievous grin. "Hello, stranger."

"Is it too soon?" he asked, his voice wobbling.

Slowly, Eunny's eyebrows went up, her grin sliding into a smirk.

"We didn't, um... I can always come back later," he said, voice tapering off.

She was dressed simply in the long yellow tunic vest she favored worn over a plain linen skirt. In the room beyond, Ollas glimpsed her things scattered about in a manner that suggested she'd abandoned unpacking midway through the process. Her tea apparatus was scattered across a countertop, next to the

water propagation glasses with a few cuttings from the delegation plants. Otherwise, the room was mild chaos.

Stepping closer, Eunny reclaimed his full attention as her
hand wrapped around the front of his shirt. She pulled him
down to kiss him, tongue darting out to tease his lips. His
mouth moved of its own volition, reaching, but she drew back.
"Oh, I'm sorry," she said, voice going husky. "You were saying
something about leaving?"

"Not anymore."

"That's what I thought."

Eunny backed up a step, then another, head tilting to the
side in silent question. Ollas followed, kicking the door shut
behind him. His boots joined hers beside the door. The cloak
went next, Ollas pausing long enough to remove the plain
mercantile bag.

The unmistakable jingle of the glass bottles inside sounded
loud in the quiet. Eunny's new lodging was a cozy single, the
design open but with plenty of space-conscious storage
options. She sat on her bed, leaning back on her hands as she
watched him. Thanks to the drawers built into the bed frame,
her feet didn't touch the ground.

Perfect. He was easily half a head taller than her; nice to
know he wouldn't have to break his back to fuck her bent over
the side.

The thought had him stiffening. Made his trousers feel
tight. Constricting.

Eunny's gaze dipped down, eyes crinkling at the corners as
her lips curved ever upward. "Did you bring me something?"
She pointed with her chin toward the bag clutched in his hand.

A self-conscious laugh bubbled up as Ollas pulled the cloth
sides down to reveal the upper halves of the vials. All four of
them.

Eunny snorted. "You planning to move in?"

"No, I-I wasn't— I didn't know if, if I should—" Ollas's hand shook as he tried to cover the bottles again, knocking one over in the process.

"I'm kidding. Give 'em here." Eunny held out her hands.

Red-faced, Ollas handed her the bag.

She made an appreciative sound as she surveyed the labels. "My favorite kind of housewarming gift." Her eyes cut back to him. Swept up and down, taking the measure of him. "Maybe my second favorite."

"Maybe?" Ollas went to his knees in front of her.

"Too soon to tell." Eunny caressed him with her bare foot. "You do look good down there."

She popped the cork on the closest vial and downed it before tossing the glass aside.

A tremor ran through his hands as he lifted them toward her legs. Her skin was warm. Soft. Ollas let his fingers skim along her calves, hesitant. He met her eyes. "Offerings for my goddess."

She laughed, scooting up enough to push the skirt off her hips. The fabric pooled at his knees. Bare flesh greeted him.

At his surprised look, Eunny shrugged one shoulder. "I figured you were coming by." Her foot hooked beneath his arm, pulled him a touch closer. "I hoped you would."

The final vestiges of trepidation, of so many years filled with yearning and doubt, fell away. Awe and relief rushed up to take their place. And hunger—so much of that.

Ollas put his lips to her calf, her knee, her thigh. Lingered there, kissing her tender skin as he inhaled. She was intoxicating. Her scent alone made a quiet groan rumble deep in his chest.

"Is this how Little Nev prayed at the Altar of Song?" Eunny teased, her eyes intent on him.

"I was a boy then." Ollas wrapped his arms around her

thighs. Pulled her closer. Parted her with his thumbs and nearly died to find her already damp at her center for him. "Tonight, I'll worship you as a man."

Her amused response cut off in a gasp the moment his mouth touched her. *Touched* being a relative word. Technically true, but ever so inadequate. Too gentle a word for what Ollas did with his tongue. He buried his face in her pussy, tongue sweeping in as far as humanly possible. Ignored her choked screech when his beard tickled her thighs. He made love to her with his mouth, a wet groan escaping when she fluttered around his tongue.

Imagination paled in comparison to the real thing. She was so soft, the heady musk of her filling his lungs. And the taste, a sweetened tang that beckoned him to come back for more. Drink his fill. He indulged, licking and sucking and stroking, spurred on by her garble of words. The occasional "fuck" and "Nev" were the only ones coherent amongst her mess.

She'd been waiting for him, pussy bare beneath her skirt. Was probably bare under her vest, too, nipples ready for his lips. Ollas was torn between checking and continuing to slowly devour her whole. To have her perfect body laid out before him. He'd watch his cock disappear inside her, see her face when she came.

Ollas moaned at the thought. Soon, but not yet. They were here, in her new, private room. No interruptions. And, as she'd said, she would need to be prepared. A task he was fully committed to delighting in.

He leaned back, wiping her desire from his face with the back of his hand. He stilled, eyes locked on the glisten of it on his skin. He licked it clean. She'd called him an animal; might as well earn it.

Eunny's head had dropped back during his attentions. Now,

she dragged it up enough to see him, her lips parted. "Gods all break, Nev."

"Tell me what you like." He kissed the inside of her knee. "What you want."

She pushed up to sitting and plucked at his shoulder. "I want you. Inside."

Ollas smiled, his cock straining against his trousers. "Not yet. Prepared, remember?"

Eunny scoffed. "I think I can handle y— *Oh.*" She moaned as he breached her entrance with two fingers. "Okay. Yes, that's good, too."

He lowered his mouth to her again. Let his fingers explore deeper, applying his tongue again as he saw fit. Eunny squirmed, encouraging and guiding with sounds and pressure. When he found a particular spot along her front wall, she clenched like she was trying to break his fingers.

Ollas huffed in amusement when she whined and twitched from where his beard tickled her sensitive skin. His tongue swirled around her clit as he slid out to stroke through her damp folds, teasing her with just the tips of his fingers before delving inside again. He massaged along her front wall, felt the way it gave beneath his touch. Rubbed the spot that made her toes clamp together. He pressed a little harder, a little faster, when Eunny tensed. Her feet flexed, legs beginning to tremble. Her breathing was growing ragged, small sounds that weren't quite full moans coloring every exhale. Ollas kept his pace and pressure steady when her fingers tangled in his hair and pulled. She wound tighter and tighter, thighs beginning to quake.

Ollas pursed his lips around her clit and sucked.

Eunny came with a cry, hips bucking into his mouth, grinding against him as her desire soaked his beard. The scent and taste of her was enough that it would've sent him over the edge if he didn't hold himself back. It was a near thing. Only the promise of being buried in her warmth for the first time kept him in check.

A pleasant tingling filtered through his subconscious, buzzing under his skin. Ollas drew out every shudder and contraction, fingers gentler now, until Eunny let herself flop onto the bed. A languid smile curled her lips. She inhaled as if to speak, then merely closed her eyes and shook her head, making only a contented purr-like sound instead.

Ollas wiped his face. Again. The thought made him grin. "I humbly serve."

"As I recall, there's nothing humble about what you've got." Eunny dragged herself upright, shucking off her vest. "Show me."

As he'd suspected, her bare breasts greeted him, her dusky pink nipples already firmed into points.

She tapped him with her foot. "Ogle *and* strip."

Ollas stood, happy to oblige. Once freed, his cock bobbed up, jutting toward his belly. Eunny reached for him, tracing his length with one finger. Wrapped her hand around him, squeezing when his eyes fluttered closed. She gave an experimental pump.

Ollas groaned. "Easy. It—it's not going to take much." He hoped the evening light hid his blush.

Eunny smeared her thumb in the fluid already leaking from his tip. "Then we should see if it'll fit." She licked her thumb clean.

Ollas was already moving before she could smirk up at him. His hands hooked behind her knees, sliding her across the mattress until her ass was just starting to dangle over the edge. He kissed each of her legs as he directed them over his shoulders, then grabbed the bottle of lubricant and uncapped it with his teeth.

"Tell me if I need to slow down," he said, lining up his cock with her entrance. "If it's too much."

Eunny's hands dug into the edge of the mattress. "Make me scream, Nev."

If Ollas wasn't already tunnel-visioned, so amped up that his brain was doing very little thinking at all, he'd have complained. Good-naturedly, but truly, it wasn't fair that she had him so thoroughly by the balls. Wasn't fair that he would've done anything for her. And so to be asked—no, *ordered*—to do such a thing, well, fuck.

His first thrust made her gasp, and she'd only taken about half of him. The second had her curling off the bed, one hand coming up to clutch his wrist.

Ollas held her by the hips. Held her close as he slowly drew back, then snapped his pelvis flush. He leaned forward to swallow down her scream. Kissed her roughly, tasting a hint of his saltiness along with traces of strawberries. So, that had been the vial she'd picked. He'd never think of the berry the same way again.

There wasn't anything gentle or fluid about his movements. Nothing sweet or slow, the kind of intimacy one might call *love-making*. Ollas plunged in and out, up to the hilt. The slap of slickened flesh hitting flesh was topped only by the pitch of Eunny's cries.

True to his word, Ollas didn't take long. Came with a bellow, Eunny held half off the bed so he could slide deep. Just when he thought his cock was spent, she reached for her clit, rubbed a frenzy of tight circles as she clenched around him, back arching even more. The pleasant buzz under his skin intensified, made his grip tighten. He could've sworn there was something electric in the air, swirling around them. A pulling sensation emanating from Eunny herself, on some innate level. Judging by the way she grasped the back of his neck, pulling him down onto her, mouths crashing together, she felt it, too.

Her orgasm proved he still had a few spurts left to give.

They collapsed onto the bed, panting for breath. For a few minutes, neither spoke, content to lie beside each other, Eunny's head tucked against his chest.

Ollas let his hand run down her arm. Settled it around her. Eunny let out a soft, blissful sigh and wiggled around so she was propped atop his chest, hand in her chin as she grinned down at him.

"That was fun." She cupped his cheek with her free hand. "You, sir, have everyone fooled."

"How so?" he mumbled, peering up at her through half-lidded eyes.

"Mild-mannered Ollas Nevin. The awkward little bean." Eunny rubbed her finger across his lip, baring her teeth in a smile when he nibbled at her. "Awkward, maybe. Mild, eh, in the daytime. But little?" She brought her leg up to nudge his deflated cock with her knee. "Not even close."

Perhaps Little Nev wasn't so tired and spent after all.

Eunny noticed, laughter in her eyes as she stroked him. She looked... radiant.

"I love seeing you like this," he said, voice soft as he reached up to cup her cheek.

She leaned into his touch. "Like what?"

"Happy. Light," he said. "It seemed like you always had a bit of sadness after... It doesn't matter. Thank you."

Eunny's eyes narrowed slightly, the beginnings of a frown creeping in.

"I've dreamed about this forever." Ollas shook his head, a faint smile on his face. "Having you here with me."

For a long moment, she didn't answer, her expression unreadable. Ollas feared he'd overstepped, finally fucked things up beyond repair. Was just starting to look for his discarded clothing when Eunny made a soft "hmph" sound.

"I am here," she said, fingers tracing across his face. "But, no labels, okay? Those only spoil the fun."

"My goddess." He kissed her fingers. "I won't give that one up."

She sat up. "So, again?" A smile slid back onto her face, this time with a wicked edge. "I think I should try sitting on my throne."

Chapter Sixteen

DAWN WAS an hour where Eunny would rather burst into flames than be awake. For reasons unbeknownst to her, Ollas apparently rose early and *liked it.* She could only assume all of the greenhouse vapors had messed with his head. She did little more than grumble and steal his warmer side of the bed when he got up, then made an equally unintelligible sound when he kissed her cheek. Whatever he murmured in her ear, Eunny was too deeply entrenched in sleep to make sense of it. She didn't hear the door close behind him.

Which was probably for the best. When she finally roused a few hours later and dragged herself to the bathhouse, Eunny reflected on the turn of events. If Ollas had still been in her bed when she'd woken, she'd have been tempted to get back on the horse. To indulge herself with his toe-curling touch. Someone had taught the shy little plant boy well. He might not have had much magic, but she wouldn't have known it from the way his fingers made her skin sing. So, yes, for the sake of her doing anything productive with her day, it was a good thing Ollas had left first. Eunny didn't possess the deep inner strength to leave her bed with him still in it. Not without making sure the previous night hadn't been a fluke.

However, a body could use a teeny bit of a break. Hard to say no to such enthusiastic attention in the moment, and Eunny had every intention of exploring Ollas as thoroughly as he'd done with her, but distance gave her a moment of clarity.

Distance also offered a chance for perspective. Her new room didn't have any food in it yet, and she owed her auntie a visit. Wrapping herself in her cloak against the light drizzle, Eunny set out for Sylvan.

It had been a good night. No denying that part. Ollas might give the impression of a bookish, mild-mannered nerd in the halls, but in bed, he'd earned her dubbing him an animal. A thoughtful, generous one, as evidenced by the pack of contraceptive potions he'd brought. Top shelf ones, too, none of the medicinal-tasting freebie ones. And he'd been so endearingly awkward about it. Shy but eager. Just the way she liked him.

Things would be different between them now. Hard for them not to be. Sleeping together had a way of doing that, especially since their whatever-it-was-between-them was so poorly defined. Eunny hadn't invested in any relationship that could be considered more than casual since her Initiate levels. Hadn't wanted a commitment. She still didn't, not really. But this thing with Ollas? She had a feeling he'd want more than casual.

I've dreamed about this forever.

Apparently, being with her hadn't doused the torch he'd been carrying. It made her feel more than a tad smug; nice not to be overhyped. But he'd want labels for whatever they were to each other. Eventually. To *have her* with him. To be hers in return.

A possessive curl rose in Eunny's chest at the thought. They both seemed amenable to the sex part, at any rate. That, she could do. Have a fling, nothing more. Nothing too serious, with announcements of intentions and publicity and telling all their friends. Nothing that would develop *feelings*. Didn't mean she had to share him, and she had a feeling Ollas wouldn't find that limiting at all.

He saw the darkness in her—the sadness, he called it. The bitterness that lingered despite the years since the delegation's end. He saw that in her, and still wanted to be a part of letting some light back in. Even though she'd broken him beyond repair. The sentiment should've hardened her resolve, intensified her guilt. It shouldn't make her breathe an inner sigh of relief.

Eunny bit the inside of her lip. Hard. *No getting soft, Eun,* she thought as a copper-tasting hint of blood crept across her tongue.

She was glad Ollas forgave her, but Eunny wouldn't be so kind. Not to herself. Not completely. She could ignore her inner critic enough to fool around with him, convince herself it was okay so long as this was just for fun. But she would not let their play become something real. She was already changing because of Ollas. A little, tiny bit. Letting her guard down. Being tempted to do things like trust, and care. To be willing to try and make not merely peace but *amends* with her magic.

Such a notion should've been unthinkable. Yet anger, once a near-constant companion, was proving harder to grasp. Ollas was just so...sweet. Good. She'd never really cared for such traits in a lover, but in him, she found it appealing.

"Couldn't say you were just trying to save me, eh, Nev?" she muttered to herself as she entered the Mighty Leaf. If he'd been on some personal mission to save her broken soul, then Eunny could've dismissed the silly feelings she was having. Probably wouldn't be at risk of growing them at all; she was no one's charity case. But he had to go and thank her, look at her all tender. Like she really was a goddess. A minor deity, perhaps, but the only one in his world. It made her feel…light. Maybe a touch happy, too.

Gods all break. She would *not* turn into a sap. They'd have their fun for now, so long as she could keep things under control. No deep feelings, no letting herself think that everything could be all right. No pretending that she could forget the harm her magic had caused, or be convinced that perhaps it wasn't so bad. Once she found herself slipping down that slope, Eunny would have to end it. For both their sakes.

She made her way to the back of the tearoom, hugging Yerina before her aunt bustled off to attend to a fresh batch of pastries. Intent on snagging her favorite corner booth, Eunny nearly passed a blond man sitting alone in a window seat, when she happened to glance down.

"Professor Sor'vahl?"

Garethe Sor'vahl glanced up from the paper he was reading. He smiled wide, laugh lines forming at the corners of his eyes. "Garethe, please. It's Miss Song, right?"

"Eunny's fine."

"Eunny, yes, you're Dae's friend. And Yerina's niece," he said with a small nod. He gestured to the open seat across from him. "Would you like to join me?"

"If I'm not interrupting?"

At his encouraging nod, Eunny sat. They chatted amiably about the shop and Eunny's admittedly indeterminate plans for the repair café.

"I do hope you get it all sorted soon," Garethe said. "It's a wonderful concept. The town loves it, from what I've seen. I'm tempted to steal the idea for back home, but I'm afraid I'm not at all handy."

"Are you going back to Rhell for the spring?"

"No, I'm committed here for the full year. Perhaps longer, depending on how things are up there." Garethe smiled, but there was a weariness about him, the lines on his face no longer full of good humor. Though he had a healthy pallor, Garethe had a gauntness to his frame that spoke of his long illness from Rhell's poison.

"So, you're assisting with Saren's elective. Fancy yourself a grovetender now?"

Eunny made a face. "Hardly." She hesitated, surreptitiously scanning the room. The Mighty Leaf always did steady business, and today was no different. Fortunately, Garethe's table was situated such that, between a knee wall directing the pathing through the room and a nearby water feature, they had a decent amount of space between them and the nearest occupied table.

Garethe leaned closer, a roguish gleam putting new vigor in his eye. "I'm already intrigued."

"It's sort of a personal question," Eunny said in apologetic tones.

He tsked at her. "I'm a terrible Rhellian. Corrupted by my time away. Ask."

Eunny thought back on the snippets of an idea that had been floating through her head. The Healing Hut, and Dae taking a healing draught imbued with her own magic. Zhenya's comment about the elective's seedlings being more potent if grown in Rhell's soil. The secret delegation plants being triggered to bloom after absorbing her magic—healing magic.

"What does the poison feel like?" she asked, voice low. "No, I guess I mean, what does the mending part after feel like?"

Garethe frowned, gaze going distant as he thought. "Exhausting. Maybe all mending feels that way to some extent.

But with a wound, you can feel a bit of *yourself* in the repair. Feel your body holding on to the magic. The poison can't be held, it only drains. It never feels like it's fully gone, either." He gave her a crooked smile. "Even here in the Valley, I can feel its touch. The Valley's is just... stronger. When I breathe in, it's like I feel the air here *stick* to me, but it's only a coating over the poison, or the illness. A cap, but it can be worn away."

"Like a dry spot in your throat?"

"If you like." A laugh sounded through his nose. "Only instead of an itch or the need to cough, it's like being stabbed. And *then* you cough, but it's to bring up blood."

"Lovely." Eunny grimaced. She traced a filled-in crack on the tabletop with her finger, her words coming out hesitant. "The treatment Dae got while she was here, the preventative? They can't make something like that for you?"

"Perhaps if I was magic-born, but I don't have anything to grant it sticking power." Garethe sat up, warmth in his manner. "Just means I get to stay down here more. It's much nicer to be in a classroom than at court, let me tell you." He stood, stretching out his back. "Speaking of, I should get back to grading, but it was a pleasure, Eunny. If you have any other questions, you're always welcome to ask."

"Thanks for indulging me." Eunny felt her grin widen. "Make those kids earn their marks."

Garethe tipped his head back with a shout of a laugh. "Not a problem from me. Poor lambs get quite the shock. They think the jolly Rhellian will be a breeze." He winked. "It's all misdirection. Sare is the soft touch, but these dear little Ini Ones are scared of him. They'll learn in time."

With a final wave, Garethe departed. Eunny watched him go, sipping at her tea as she tried to reconcile the cheerful Rhellian man with the reserved, stately Professor Rai. An unlikely pairing, but then, she was one to talk. Appearances could be deceiving, after all. As recently as a few weeks ago, Eunny wouldn't have believed she'd be sleeping with Ollas Nevin. Would've laughed at the very thought.

Yerina took Garethe's vacated seat, setting a small plate of fresh teacakes in front of Eunny. "New batch of red beans and Deiju syrup just came in this morning."

Eunny bit into one, a gratified moan vibrating in her throat. "So good. Thanks, Auntie. Sorry I haven't been by lately."

"I can manage without you, Eunny dear. It's good for you to be out." Yerina watched Eunny wolf down another teacake. "I saw Gransen going through the café earlier."

"Didn't waste time, did he?" Eunny snorted. "I'm surprised he didn't just camp out there."

"You've decided on repairs?"

"I've delegated."

A smile filled Yerina's face. "I'm glad. The town just doesn't feel right with it closed."

Eunny's own smile felt weak at the edges, as it always did when her repair café and the concept of permanency came up. She loved her aunt, but someone so kindly and full of sunshine would never understand the reticence Eunny felt. The guilt and the wrongness, trying to insert herself into the community like she was one of them. As if she deserved to be there despite what her rogue magic had done. Finding a level of personal comfort in the Grove was one thing, but having a space in the heart of Sylvan still made unease prickle her skin. To Yerina and her eternal optimism, those kinds of thoughts just didn't register. The town loved her and tolerated Eunny sliding in on her auntie's cloak tails. Eunny wasn't foolish enough to hope for anything more. Would never ask for it.

Yerina didn't notice Eunny's frozen expression, but it was just as well, for she moved on to easier topics. "Tell me about your new work. How is Ollas doing? Terryl said he was almost recovered when she was in last week."

Eunny chuckled. Her aunt rarely set foot on the campus grounds, but being good friends with Ollas's mother, Terryl Nevin, a reference librarian at the school, ensured she was well informed on any school gossip.

She regaled her aunt with stories from the elective and Eunny's middling attempts to grow the same plants as the class. Though she kept the specifics of her dabbling in apothecary work to a minimum, she admitted to enjoying being back at the school, and to her decision to linger until she was formally kicked out.

"It's still mostly hauling dirt and stuff back and forth, cleaning pots and tools, that sort of thing. But... I like it," Eunny said. "It's different being there, this time around. The approach. It's all new."

"I'm sure. You could barely keep my window boxes alive, let alone study like an earth mage." Yerina chortled to herself as she got to her feet. "Oh, before I forget, you've got a letter from Dae. I was just about to have it sent up to the school."

She dug around in an apron pocket and pulled out a small envelope with Dae's clean handwriting on the front.

"I'll tell your mother about your school adventures in my next letter," Yerina said, her tone becoming too casual. Eunny suppressed the urge to roll her eyes. "Unless you'd rather tell her yourself?"

"Only you enjoy one-way correspondence, Auntie," Eunny said dryly. "Tell her. Don't tell her. She's not going to care either way."

In typical Yerina fashion, she managed to both ignore Eunny's negativity and insist she was wrong at the same time. She hugged her again before going back to checking on patrons, and Eunny made her way back to Sylveren.

Her aunt's joy in Eunny's activities reminded her of Ollas—happy that she seemed happy. And Eunny *was*. More than she could remember being in a long while. Unburdened enough that she'd actually touched her magic, even if by accident. Only a touch, but even that would've been unthinkable at the start of term. She'd drawn up a few drops of magic and it had been... fine.

Eunny read Dae's letter as she made her way back to the Grove. Considering they'd just seen each other in the last fortnight, Dae must have written it shortly after arriving back in Rhell. Eunny knew they liked to correspond a lot, but this was excessive.

Dae's letter was indeed short. Not even a proper letter-letter, but more like a hastily penned note. The secret delegation plant had transplanted well into the containment zone's blighted soil, and preliminary tests from the camp's mender suggested it would apply well to preventative tonics. Not enough to cure those badly sickened by long exposure to the poison, but effective in slowing the concentrated toxicity's ability to infect the healthy.

The menders think this might eliminate the need to leave the containment zones for long periods to recuperate, Dae wrote. *Make more if you can!*

Eunny reread Dae's final plea, the words burning into memory long after she'd stowed the note back in her cloak pocket.

Maybe Ollas was right. The secret plants' rate of change seemed to support his theory. The strange pull. The restlessness that had been building all summer, that had taken off once Eunny and Ollas were in close proximity again, once the plants had gotten a taste of her magic. Could the medley of sensations all have been part of the imprinting spell he spoke of, imparting a subconscious urge to fulfill it? To make the plants bloom? But they fed on magic—her magic—and they needed more of it to make it past the current stall they had at just leaves. Ollas could propagate every single clump outside of the greenhouse, but they wouldn't achieve their new state, the healing variety Dae wrote of, without magic.

Back in her new apartment, Eunny immediately went to the counter where her trio of stems were suspended in glass vials filled with plain water. They'd exploded with new roots overnight. When she brought her face up next to one, a faint pulse of warmth emanated from the leaves.

Hesitantly, she touched one of the leaves and called up just a speck of her inner light. Only a scrap of it, enough to search for a hint of resonance and no more.

A single sparkle of golden light slipped from her finger to the satiny green leaf. It flared bright like an ember, then winked out. Yet in that brief moment, Eunny felt a hum of magic, as if the plant had been imbued. The hum held familiar notes of her own magic...and something else. Some*one* else.

Not body magic, but she'd remember the signature of Ollas and his thready light forever. Would always remember how her magic had ensnared him, tangled with his feeble light and traced through his body, wreaking havoc.

I think it's us.

The memory of their electric lovemaking dimmed a bit in Eunny's mind. He was right; they *were* affecting the plants. The imprinting spell, or whatever caused the instinctive pull in them, it took advantage when passions were running high. Any time self-control waned.

Eunny sank into a chair, eyes never leaving the plants in their glass vials on the counter. They were still so small. Now that she looked at them and knew their inner hum, it was impossible not to feel it: a gentle presence but persistent, always tugging for more. She hadn't been able to put a name to the feeling before, but now...

The idea of giving the plants more of herself was disquieting. Had needles of fear and denial and *no* clamoring in her head. She balled her hands into fists, fingernails biting into her palms enough to make the rising panic subside. The pain didn't vanish fully, but it gave her enough room for clarity.

She wasn't in this alone.

Chapter Seventeen

Nevin—Sorry this took so long, but I had to hunt just for this much. Noc Lowe is liaising with the Coalition for waterway access, might know someone who knows more. Let me know if you want to get in touch.

OLLAS'S FRIEND who clerked for the Sentinels had finally written back. If one could call this brief letter such; it was attached to a hasty copy of the Sentinel inventory logs. Many items were scratched or blacked out, with a scribble at the bottom indicating transfer to an unintelligible name. A jaggedness to the magicked pigment used for the copying work implied that parts of the logs had been torn away. At the end of the last page was a weak impression of the Coalition's seal of a wheel enclosing a coin.

He didn't have a lot of hope that Ranger Noc Lowe could get any more news if the Coalition was involved, but anything was better than the pages of heavily redacted records.

Frowning at the sorry state of the "logs," Ollas went into the storage greenhouse to check on the new tray of cuttings started from the delegation plants. He knelt to observe them where they were stowed on the lower shelf. All but one had fully converted from resembling grass to bearing blade-shaped leaves. Further inspection revealed that the lone outlier wasn't simply slower to change than its brethren—it had died.

Removing the dead plant from the tray, Ollas carried the pot back into the greenhouse's main room. He left the pot in the washbasin to be cleaned later and carried what remained of the plant over to the counter, stopping short of the compost collection bucket. A physical inspection didn't reveal any signs of rot or disease, no pest infestation or anything else that would indicate a need for the burn pile. But there was also nothing that would easily explain why the plant had turned a deadish brown and gone crispy, as if it had dried out. The soil around the brittle roots remained moderately wet. A quick test with one of the soil probes reported good parameters, which were echoed when he checked the surviving starts, too.

A frown creased his brow. Ollas never expected a perfect success rate, and sometimes an individual simply didn't thrive. But seedling death didn't usually appear so at odds with the growing conditions. His failed plantlet looked as if it had been dehydrated.

Ollas summoned a touch of his magic and gently pushed it into a browned leaf. The plant didn't absorb his magic so much as the drop of golden light shattered, breaking apart into the tiniest wisp of smoke and fading away.

"What happened to you?" Ollas murmured.

"Nev!"

Ollas turned to the greenhouse door, a smile already spreading across his face as he looked for her. Eunny came in, a glass jar from her water propagation setup in one hand. She set the jar on the counter, bumping her hip against his side before letting an innocent amount of space form between them.

Ollas cupped her cheek and went in for a kiss. Happiness zipped through him from head to groin when Eunny's tongue darted out to tease his lips before she pulled back.

She pouted at him. "You get up too early."

"Creature of habit. Got to be up with the sun."

Eunny huffed a laugh. "Well, *Professor,* fancy some more experimentation?"

He'd rather do more experimentation of her, but there'd be time for that later. He made a noise of pleasant surprise when she showed him the explosive growth of her cutting. "This is amazing. Did you add something else to the water?"

"Nope. As you said, I guess they like us."

Ollas gave her a quizzical look. She spoke in a light tone, but there was something veiled in her expression. He looked from her to the plant. "You mean, from us...sleeping together?"

"Or they just really like my new place," she said. "Ever hear of that for imprinting enchantments?"

"No, proximity alone shouldn't be enough to satisfy the spellwork," Ollas muttered, more to himself than Eunny. He gestured to the dead plant he'd set on the counter. "Nothing about these has been typical or ordinary, though."

Eunny glowered at it. "Unacceptable. You want for nothing. All the food and water a plant could ask for. Get to live all cozy inside. The least you could do is grow."

"To be fair, they're doing that part really well," Ollas said. "One failure in—"

She transferred her glare from the plant to him. "Don't excuse their malicious compliance."

"They're plants, Eunny, they don't have malice." Ollas paused, mouth twisting. "*Most* don't. None that we'd grow in the school's greenhouses do, anyway." He edged away, reached into his pocket, and withdrew a sealed jar with a tiny brush attached to the lid. Uncapping it, he dabbed a light green powder onto the dry, flaky parts of the old vines that hung around the antechamber's windows.

"Appeasing our future floral overlords?" Eunny teased.

Ollas shrugged. Trunk wasn't a hotbed of activity, of either the magical or mundane sort. Hard to say if the aged resident protection plant retained any of those instincts or if it had gradually lost them as it went creaky with age. But, he figured it was better to be safe than sorry. "We could always conduct more research. See if we can get the cuttings to grow more."

She laughed. "Oh, Nev, I intend to." His cock stirred in response to the way her voice lowered. "However," she continued, "I'd rather you have my full attention, and in the meantime, I've heard back from Dae about the baby plant she took home. Transplanted like a champ, and it has healing properties."

"Really?" Ollas grabbed the notebook where he was keeping a record of the delegation plant experiments. "Did she say what the growing conditions are?"

"It was a short note, but I know it's planted in contaminated dirt," Eunny said. "Strong preventative qualities, not a cure."

He copied down her words. "More than what I got back from the Sentinels, though that's not really their fault." He pointed to where the redacted logs sat on the counter. "We might be on our own for this. I've got another contact to try, but..."

Eunny perused the papers, which were more blackened bars and scratches than words. She let out a low whistle. "You weren't kidding. Oh, great, more Coalition fuckery. Guess I shouldn't be surprised that they inserted themselves, since they were part of the delegation, but this is ridiculous. What do you need to censor in a report about a failed trade delegation? Aside from them failing, I guess, but that's a moot point."

"The Sentinels have a ranger working with the Coalition now. Maybe he'll have better luck. But in the meantime"—Ollas gestured with his pencil toward her rooted cutting—"we have a shipment of soil from a containment zone. Want to try potting this up?"

"Sure. Need me to grab anything special?"

"The amendments the elective is using for the healing trial. Time to see if our theory about these plants wanting light magic holds up."

Eunny left to gather the requisite materials from the Adept levels' greenhouse while Ollas retrieved one of the enchanted terrariums being used to house smaller amounts of Rhell's blighted soil.

When they met back up in Trunk, Eunny lifted her cutting. "Can I do the planting?"

"Of course." Ollas offered her a pair of gloves, but she shook her head.

"I want to feel the *soil,* like a proper grovetender. I'll be quick, promise."

He hesitated. "Is that wise?" Even though the contact would be brief and they were in the Valley, the thought of her unprotected skin touching the corrupt ground made his hands shake with the urge to snatch her away.

"I won't tell if you don't." She flashed him a quick smile, though her eyes remained tense. "Talk me through this again."

He did, instructing her on combining amendment with the corrupted soil mix and the depth of the hole to make, reminding her to keep a light touch when firming the soil around the roots and stem of her cutting. He poured a small amount of accelerant into the terrarium and gave her a fresh stirring rod, advising that she fluff the area around the stem.

Eunny nodded along, eyes glued to her task. Her bare finger swirled through the soil, her expression serious. "Tell me the timeframe we're looking at again?"

"This is all guesswork," Ollas said. "But if it goes as well as it did for Anadae, we could see changes by tomorrow. Morning, if it's really fast."

He watched Eunny, noting the tightness in her features. The fine sheen of sweat forming on her brow.

At the edge of his mind, he felt a slight tug of awareness. Of recognition. Of *magic.*

He went still, but Eunny was too consumed with her task to notice. Magic. That brush against his senses, weak as it was, weak as *his* magic was, couldn't be denied. Ollas wasn't a powerful mage, but he could recognize the arcane. Had enough ability to identify the essence of magic, if not the signature, and what he felt now wasn't from any branch he knew. Which made sense; Eunny wasn't an elementalist at all.

He was feeling Eunny's light. Something hazy in the back of his mind warmed at the familiarity. Slowly, he made the connection to the buzzy feeling when they'd had sex, the sparking sensations between their skin. At the time, he'd been so enthralled with being with Eunny that he hadn't done any critical thinking. But as he tried to grasp the details steeped in euphoria, deeper memories stirred. Ones that didn't have the same blissful glow. Their magic intertwining—he'd felt that before, too. Ever so briefly, before everything went horribly wrong.

"Nev."

Eunny's voice broke Ollas from his musing.

"Keep talking," she said without looking up. "Just, uh, keep my mind off the fact that I'm wrist-deep in poisoned dirt."

"Sure. Um." He fought to keep his voice calm. Level. Unsuspecting. "We did something like this for my Adept Two research."

He blathered on about cold, wet nights in the mountains. Meanwhile, his mind whirred over this revelation. Eunny had her magic, in some amount. He couldn't be sure if she was using it consciously or if some part of the process drew it from her unbeknownst to Eunny herself. He didn't dare to ask. Not with how adamantly she professed to be against using it.

If this was a subconscious awakening of her threads of magic, then he'd need to tread softly. At least until she warmed to the notion of having magic again. Ollas would be at her side regardless.

"Done." Eunny slapped the rod down with a triumphant look. She closed the glass roof panel on the box. "Is this going to fit on the shelf?"

It took some rearranging, but they managed to create space to hide their secret project away again. She gave him a quick kiss. "Thanks."

"Eunny..." He started to speak but couldn't get further than her name. Where to begin? "We should... You—"

She covered his mouth with her hand. "Not yet. Not *no*, just not *yet*. Can't we just enjoy how things are for a bit before we make decisions?"

Bad idea. Delaying such conversations, not knowing where they really stood? Definitely a bad, bad idea. He was grown enough to know better, but when his mouth opened again, all that came out was, "Sure."

"Good. Anything else we can do for that?" Eunny nodded with her chin at the terrarium. "Waiting isn't really my strong suit."

Ollas rubbed his chin. "Zhenya might be able to help."

"What'll ink do?"

"I was thinking more of how she tends to know at least a

little about everything botanical," Ollas said with a short laugh. "She's already looked into the similarities with rare blooming varieties, and she's more familiar with imprinting spells than I am, at least the theory behind the workings. Not sure how recently that was, but..." He shrugged.

Eunny mimicked the motion. "I'll see if I can find her."

He checked the wall clock. "My guess is the library. I'll go with you."

"Don't you have a report due to the Restorers?" Her nose wrinkled. "And my mother."

He held the door open for her. "It can wait. The second trial's been lagging this week, anyway. If she doesn't believe me, she can come out and see for herself."

The library at Sylveren University was a grand building, all aged wood, though it was comprised of so much glass it was more window than wall. Large trees flanked the multilevel building, stalwart evergreens rather than the ethereal maple that was the Grove. Some kind of vine climbed up the front of the building near the main entrance. It appeared as if the vine had been meant to frame the large double doors as a decorative element—Eunny had a vague recollection of there being pretty, papery flowers as big as her fist during the summer—but now, the vine was nearly leafless for the approaching winter, and it had escaped containment, sending out branches in all directions.

Eunny followed Ollas up to the second level reference desk. His step faltered as they approached the older woman seated there.

"Hello, Ma," he said. "Have you seen Zhenya around?"

Though the question was spoken cordially enough, there was a note of warning in his tone.

"Olly! I wasn't ex—" Terryl Nevin looked up, her eyes widening with delight when she noticed— "Eunny! What are you doing here?"

"Zhenya, Ma. Looking for Zhenya," Ollas said, stooping down to kiss his mother's cheek. The family resemblance was strong, from their dark curls to their full faces, though Terryl's hair was more gray than brown, now, and her cheeks hollowed with age. But they had the same smile, the same laugh.

There was something endearing about the picture they made, but it carried with it a sense of melancholy, too, and Eunny couldn't have said why.

"Stacks, red corner. Something about murals." Terryl smiled at Eunny. "I haven't seen you up in these parts in ages."

True. Eunny hadn't set foot in the library since her Initiate-level days. She'd done some repair work for different sections, but the materials came to her, usually by way of Zhenya. Still, Terryl herself was hardly a stranger, being Auntie Yerina's best friend and all. Eunny had known the woman since she was a kid, and saw her often enough down at the Mighty Leaf. Back when open crafting nights had still been regular events at the café, Terryl had regularly attended and helped with any sewing questions.

A pang that was more guilt than sadness hit Eunny as she ducked her head. "Guess schooling wasn't quite done with me yet." She nudged Ollas. "He's a terrible influence. Good teacher, though."

Ollas's ears went red. "We're going to find Zhen."

Eunny waved. "It was good to see you, Terryl."

"Come by any time, dear."

Leaving a grinning Terryl at her desk, they trotted off to the red corner and found Zhenya seated on the top rung of a ladder as she scribbled away in a notebook.

"I'm no expert, but this can't be safe," Eunny remarked.

"What are you doing here?" Zhenya stowed her pen and climbed down with exaggerated care.

"Looking for you. Is there, uh, some place"—Eunny glanced around—"a little more private?"

Zhenya led them to one of the empty study rooms, closing the door behind them and activating the noise ward. "Is this about your propagation experiment in Trunk?"

Eunny and Ollas exchanged looks. "You explain," Eunny said.

Ollas complied, filling in the gaps in what Zhenya already knew—or had surmised on her own from poking around their not-so-hidden tray in the storage greenhouse. Eunny supplemented his commentary as needed, admitting that her magic might well have poured out and triggered a hidden imprinting spell, if one existed in the seeds Ollas had found. She avoided mentioning that her gift was still very much present and had been fed into the delegation plants, even if in small amounts. She left the effusive comments on the nascent pull of the plants to Ollas. Neither brought up how their sleeping together might've been the catalyst for Eunny's cuttings' dramatic growth.

"You've done more with imprinted spellwork than me," Ollas said. "Does any of this sound familiar?"

"I was doing work on imbued iconography," Zhenya said. "Which is sort of related, because the inks with highest water resistance originated in the north. The methods do, at any rate."

"What does water resistance have to do with the delegation plants?" Eunny asked.

"Nothing. The *methods*. Seeds were imbued with different magics to try and influence the resulting plants with those qualities." Zhenya flipped back a dozen pages in her overstuffed notebook, scanning the contents with an ink-stained finger. She stopped, tapping a line. "The imbuing process, the sequence, it's usually done in stages. Each requires... magic."

"Magic," Eunny repeated, slowly.

Zhenya nodded. "From what I've read, and there's not much, so this is barely more than conjecture, but these imprinting sequences are a safeguard. A means to keep different properties separate, but also secure. Linked to the mage. Or mages, in your case."

"What are— I'm not an academic, Zhen. Simple words. Explain it like I'm five."

Her eyes drifted upward in thought. "I think the seeds imprinted on you. Like baby ducks. It's possible they had previously been spelled to require earth and light magic to grow, and when your, um, accident happened, you unintentionally triggered that spell."

"Okay," Eunny said weakly. "So, the plants are imprinted on us. Like ducks. Great. What does that mean?"

"Your magic bonded to the natural bit of life in each seed. But like I said, there are stages. That stored life doesn't last forever, imbued or not. You said one of your divisions died in a weird way?"

Eunny snuck a glance at Ollas. His brow was furrowed in thought, and he nodded, murmuring, "Like it had dried out. Lack of magic, instead of water?"

Zhenya nodded. "It makes the most sense. It sounds like you've woken the next stage of the imprinting sequence, the blooming period."

"Only we haven't gotten any of them to bloom," Eunny said.

Zhenya gave a small shrug. "They're going to need more magic. Presumably yours, Eunny, though I guess it's possible another source of light magic could take them over. Like calls to like, in most cases."

"Goddess fucking break," Eunny muttered. She'd already

had a suspicion, but Zhenya's confirmation didn't make her feel better for being proven right.

"Hard to say how long they'll stay in the blooming phase since we don't know what they are, but it won't wait forever," Zhenya said, worry on her face. "Sorry. I wish I had better news."

Eunny forced a smile. "Not your fault. You've been a lot of help—I mean it. Thanks, Zhen."

Leaving their friend to her research, Eunny and Ollas trudged back to the reference desk. Terryl was still there and beckoned them closer.

"Olly, there's been some questions about a paper for your Initiate One class," Terryl said. "Could you pop over and make sure Jiasi has what she needs?"

Eunny paused by the chair opposite the desk. "Is it the elective? Should I go help?"

"No, no, sit." Terryl leaned closer, her voice lowering despite their relative privacy as Ollas went to the opposite end of the room. "I want to thank you, Eunny dear, for helping out my Ollas like you did. That elective is so important to him."

"It was the least I could do. My roof *fell* on him."

Terryl dismissed Eunny's attempt at modesty with a toss of her head. "Nonsense. You don't make buildings collapse, and you put your café on hold for his work. I won't forget that, and Olly won't, either."

"It was no trouble," Eunny said, embarrassed. "I'm happy to help. The students really do seem to love him."

Terryl chuckled. "They do, and he loves it here. He's been quite happy lately."

Discomfort of an entirely different sort had Eunny blushing and stammering out, "That's—that's, well, y-you know..."

Terryl *winked* at her. "He's always been smitten with you, dear." Some of her mirth dimmed, replaced by sympathy. "He never felt right about how the delegation was handled, not for you or for him. Homegrown Hero. I'm glad my boy finally got some proper respect, but the way city folk were acting around here..." Terryl muttered to herself, gaze unfocused. She shook her head, attention back on Eunny. "Your coming here was a good thing. Never seen your auntie happier, aside from when she first took up with Dex."

"Thanks." Eunny managed a smile and stood. "I've got to run an errand. Idea from Zhen. Could you tell Ollas I'll see him in class tomorrow?"

At Terryl's bemused nod, Eunny fled. Luck was with her, and she didn't run into Ollas on her way to the door, escaping out into the rain.

Instead of following the path back to Belle, Eunny took the side road that led down to Sylvanor Lake. The vast body of water was dark and choppy from the wind and rain, its surface a mirror for the emotions roiling beneath her skin.

Ollas had been nursing a crush on her since boyhood and had finally seen it to fruition. His mother had *thanked* her for it. Thanked Eunny for making her son so happy. Because Ollas liked her. Found joy in being with her, despite all the bad her presence in his life had wrought. Wanted to save her after all.

The worst part was, he had.

Eunny bit her lip, as if the pain would make the tumult in her head become sense. Ollas had picked up on the undercurrent of anger and disillusionment and sadness she carried, and, whether wittingly or not, he'd had the impulse to *fix it*. To make it all better.

He couldn't soothe that which she had nurtured herself. Couldn't simply erase the guilt she felt—at hurting him, at losing control of her magic. Being a danger. No one like that should be allowed back into the magical community. She didn't *want* back into it. The bit of fun she was having with Ollas wasn't supposed to be serious. It was just a *fling*. She'd always intended for him to be a casual lover. Yet, now that she had to enforce those feelings on herself, where was her conviction?

Eunny was never supposed to start caring about things again. Not deeply. When faced with the quiet revelations about Ollas and his feelings, the way he offered them to her so freely, she was filled with guilt. She didn't deserve his goodness, not when she'd broken him.

Where was her old anger, her hate? That had always made it easy to rebuke the shreds of longing, of weakness, when they'd tried to grow larger in the past. It had kept her content whenever she looked out her café's window to the world beyond and seen a different life than what she'd envisioned. She had buried any sense of attachment—to anything—long ago.

He's good for you, Eunji.

She glared out at the water, waves crashing at her feet. The lake was usually a calming presence, putting her mind at ease if it couldn't provide outright answers. Being on its shores usually made her feel better. Lighter. Eunny was neither a wind nor a water mage, but she thought she felt a ghost of the latent power around her. The crackle in the air, mist hitting her face. All of it wanted to resonate with her light.

She held her hand in front of her, palm up, and watched as raindrops pattered off her skin. It would only take a single spot of light, a mere whisper of her magic, to feel the connection with this place. To feel the Valley's claim resonate with the sphere of magic at her core.

No. Eunny clenched her hand into a fist and dropped her arm back to her side. Magic was no good to her. Magic had shown *she* was not good, only dangerous. If she could slip up so badly once, what was to stop it from happening again? She couldn't. Couldn't reach out to it as if nothing had happened. Usually, she didn't have trouble remembering that part.

Ollas made her forget. Almost.

But she couldn't forget. She'd just have to remind him this was a dalliance, nothing more. Fun, yes, but ultimately meaningless. Soon enough, she'd be gone again, back to her repair café. Back to a life where she wasn't tempted to forgive her magic.

Ollas eroded those barriers of self-control, and because of that, Eunny knew they could never last.

Chapter Eighteen

FEELING TOO restless for the confines of her apartment, but not wanting to run into Ollas again just yet, Eunny made the trip into Sylvan. She hadn't had a quiet evening at the Mighty Leaf in a while, and with luck, she'd get to spend some more time with Yerina as well.

Luck wasn't with her. Though the tearoom was relatively quiet, with only a few tables and cushions occupied by customers, one such person was appearing with disturbing regularity.

"Eunji, won't you sit with me?" her mother said, gesturing to the empty chair across from her.

Eunny cast a desperate look around the room, but there were no easy escapes at hand. She considered leaving, politeness and basic human decency not being things she fretted over when it came to dealing with her mother. But then, out the corner of her eye, Eunny watched Auntie Yerina pause at the door leading to the back room. Her whole frame seemed to swell with a breath of hope, and then she was gone again. Probably to send Dex or one of the other servers out to check on the few customers, with instructions to give mother and daughter a wide berth.

Not trying to hide her lack of enthusiasm, Eunny flopped into the proffered chair. "Why are you such a bad sister to Auntie Yerina?"

"Excuse me?" Bioon said, brows rising as a condescending smile formed on her lips.

"Skipping out on the parenting thing, fine, I don't care. Best thing for us to only see each other in small doses. But Auntie Yerina tries so hard for you, for us to have some semblance of a family. You don't even write her—"

"I know you love to paint me as the villain, Eunji, but consider this: Yeri isn't some sweet, innocent being snubbed by her evil sister. Did it ever occur to you that she acts out of guilt?"

"For what?" Eunny said, her suspicion plain.

"This shop was supposed to be ours, once. She went behind my back, made it in her own vision. Is it really so surprising I don't enjoy coming here and seeing what could've been mine too?" As if remembering herself, Bioon added in a silky tone, "Ours. What we could have done together."

Eunny glanced around the Mighty Leaf, taking in its indoor water feature and the way the decor blended designs from the eastern Radiant Isles and the western influences of Graelynd and the Valley. It was warm and inviting, offering quieter nooks to relax or study along with tables and booths for those looking to be more social. A wall near the front counter offered prepackaged teas in a variety of classic favorites and more limited blends to suit any palette. The same could be said for the variety of confections and baked goods Yerina sourced from locals or made herself. One of the seasonal menus lay on the edge of their table, written and illustrated with Zhenya's color-changing inks. Everything about the shop sang of its place within the town, and of the community itself. Of personal touches and sentimentality. Bioon possessed no sense of community or sentimentality.

"Thank the Goddess she did that, then," Eunny said at last. "You really expect sympathy from me? Or belief? You couldn't be bothered to parent, so what chance did a teashop have?"

Bioon gave her a sour look. "I got you the best tutors, admission to elite schools, and work opportunities. You've turned your nose up at everything I've given you."

"Best for *you*." Eunny rolled her eyes. "*Your* idea of a model daughter, doing all the flashy, trendy shape-mending for Grae-lynd's elite. I'm not even good at that kind of detail work. How well would that have gone over when you trotted me out at parties?"

Bioon was silent for a moment, lips pursed. "I did what I could to set you up for a good life. My connections make—"

"About your *connections*," Eunny interrupted. "You want to be all involved in the elective's work? Explain to me why the Coalition went in and messed with the Sentinels' records from the delegation."

"You'll have to be more specific," Bioon murmured. "What documentation are you interested in?"

"The trade delegation. The records of what the Sentinels recovered during the rescue. I've seen the logs. They're trashed, signed by some Coalition scribble. Why sign stuff over to your-self and censor the hell out of it in the first place?"

"Likely because the delegation involved confidential terms and items beyond the purview of the Sentinels, seeing as they aren't a Graelynd institution," Bioon said with a dismissive wave of her hand. "I can't imagine what use those would be to them or you. Unless this has some bearing on the elective?"

Eunny mimed her mother's dismissive gesture. "Who can say? Hard to know when we haven't been able to read them."

"I'm sure there's nothing of consequence in the Coalition's assets."

"Oh? I seem to recall you dragging me along to assess the healing properties of plants that were part of the negotiations. And seeing as you don't have magic, is it really for you to say what is or isn't relevant to a class whose focus is to make magical plants?"

Bioon leaned forward. "So, the healing cultivar is progressing. The last reports didn't mention anything about this side research."

"We're not sure this applies to the elective. The conditions are"—Eunny shrugged—"delicate."

Her mother said nothing, but Eunny could practically see the calculations going on behind her eyes. Weighing Eunny's words against whatever information she possessed of the Coalition's dealings. Trying to decide the value in revealing more, for the Coalition gave nothing away for free.

"Delicate, you say," Bioon said. "That seems like the sort of work that would require magic. I take it yours is returning? How wonderful."

"I didn't say—"

"How else would you know that something may or may not apply to the elective?" she asked. "And you mention the appraisals you performed during the delegation. How very specific."

Her mother's smile turned Eunny's insides cold. She rallied quickly, pasting the fakest smile she could muster onto her face. "Mundanes can work with imbued materials, Mother. It's normal to feel a resonance depending on the strength of magic."

"If you say so." Bioon's voice lowered, darkening as she murmured, "You'd do well to remember that the Coalition is not to be trifled with. If there's anything you think my colleagues should know, I'm listening."

Eunny stared at her mother, both impressed with and disturbed by the way Bioon could deliver a threat with a humoring smile on her face. "Nothing comes to mind," she said.

Bioon's mouth twitched as if she were on the cusp of saying more, but then her gaze shifted. She looked past Eunny and lifted her chin in acknowledgement.

Yerina approached, eyes darting between sister and niece. "Everything all right? Bi, would you like some of the huckleberry teacakes for—"

"No, Yeri, my tastes have changed." Bioon stood up, ignoring her sister's pained look, and glanced down at Eunny. "Do tell Ollas that I expect thorough reporting if the Coalition is to entertain any record requests."

She left without waiting for a response. Probably for the best, since all Eunny came up with on the spot was mostly cursing. After chatting with her aunt for a bit, neither of them in the most talkative of moods, she trudged back toward the school. Unease itched beneath her skin as she ran through the conversation with her mother, but she couldn't pinpoint the exact cause. Bioon suspected Eunny's inquiries were for the elective, which wasn't true, but would that cause trouble for Ollas and Rai? And the way she'd hung on the notion of Eunny's returning magic... None of it boded well for Eunny being able to keep such things a secret. Especially not with Zhenya's grim revelation about the delegation plants and the ticking clock of their bloom cycle, the new problem of them starting to shrivel and die without magic.

Eunny massaged her temples. She remembered the seeds from the delegation. How they'd seemed to absorb her magic when she tested them for any innate healing properties. Had she already started the imprinting process back then? Been the seeds' first taste of magic? Despite Zhenya's theories of the plants transferring to any source of light magic, Eunny doubted the likelihood of that. Worse, a curl of possessiveness rose up at the thought of their plants, hers and Ollas's, being handed off to someone else.

"You've got to get the fuck out, Eun," she murmured to herself.

Get the plants to bloom. Make more for Dae. Then get out before she fucked up and did something absolutely unallowed... like fall for Ollas.

She'd break his sweet heart, if she had to. And all without spilling the secret of her magic.

Chapter Nineteen

THE NEXT MORNING dawned gray and misty, as was standard for deep fall in the Valley of Sylveren. Or any time for the region, the notable chill in the air being the only way to differentiate seasons. Unlike the day before, Eunny woke feeling lighter, more determined not to overthink but simply enjoy. She banished the dark cloud that always seemed to linger after an encounter with her mother—only fun allowed. Nothing serious in any regard. No dwelling on likelihoods or what-ifs. That wasn't her way; Eunny didn't look back. Forward only and leave the shit behind. It was a mindset that had been working out well for her so far. In her experience, people were happy to follow her lead. No one liked confronting uncomfortable truths if given an escape route.

Thinking she'd pop by the storage greenhouse while the main sheds were busy with Initiate classes, Eunny opened her door and nearly smacked into Gransen.

"Gremlin. Hello," she said once she'd recovered from her shock. "Can I help you?"

Gransen held up the sheaf of papers containing the estimates and options for renovating Song's Scrap. His untidy scrawl covered the pages in blue ink. "Got a moment to go over this?"

"Walk and talk." Eunny sidestepped him out onto the road. Gransen scrambled after her, shielding the papers from the light mist.

"Top page is the proposed schedule for structured fixes. Walls, roof, floors. Woodworkers' Guild thinks the floors are mostly salvageable, and they can repurpose bits from the other parts since we don't care about matching. Most of the roof and wall that came down are goners, and winter coming isn't great for repairs. It's doable, but we can get a better deal if we just go small and temporary for now and save the full job for early next year." Gransen spoke in rapid-fire sentences. "Cost is reasonable, and I've already talked with a rep at the bank about a loan."

"Gransen."

"Really reasonable rates!" He flipped a few pages. "I've drawn up some possible work schedules and new price structures to fund everything. Already got a lot of new jobs willing to pay an advance, too."

"You're already lining up work?" Eunny cried. "Gransen, I can't even start— The café is full of shit right now. It has a piece of waxed canvas for a roof! You can't go—"

"When was the last time you looked at the café?" he asked, brows raised.

"I was just..."

But she hadn't checked on Song's Scrap, only the Mighty Leaf and her auntie. Eunny all but averted her eyes when it came to her café. Still, she'd have noticed if it had grown a stable rooftop overnight. Right?

She glared at him. "It's not fit for habitation."

"Maybe not," Gransen said, "but we're not asking anyone to live there."

"You keep saying 'we,' I notice."

"You did tell me to manage. Delegated, as I recall, so, I did my job." He flipped another page with more drama than such movement required. "Now, ancillary expenses."

Eunny eyed the crude sketch in one corner. "Didn't I say no to curtains already?"

"Hear me out. The Weavers' Guild wants to do a whole workshop around them. Fluff to bolts to fabric, or whatever. Fundraise and involve the town in the process. Might even get some of the Renstownies to come over, though of course we'd charge them double."

"I don't know. This sounds like—"

"It's communal, Eun. It'll be good. Have some faith in me."

Gransen's enthusiasm, far from catching, only served to deepen the pit forming in Eunny's stomach. His ideas had merit, probably, but resistance reared its head. Filled her with a sense of refusal. Because renovations, while needed, had a ring of permanence that left her itchy with a nameless guilt. When the café had been held together with little more than waxed canvas drapes and baling twine it was easy to convince herself that she could've packed up and moved on whenever she wanted. Because Song's Scrap was a glorified popup, not a place that had put down roots and gathered a community. Those were things she didn't—couldn't—want anymore. Second chances were nice and all, but there were limits. Healers who caused egregious harm to their patients...

"I'll think about it," she said at last.

"Ok, but we—*you*—need to make some decisions soon," Gransen said. "At least let me finish with the temporary weather-sealing. The Mighty Leaf needs it so they can finish repairing the loft."

Auntie Yerina hadn't said anything about that. Eunny bit

back a sigh, nodding wearily instead. "Fine, but that's it. The rest has to wait. I'm busy with this plant stuff."

Gransen gave her a sidelong glance. "How are things with my boy?"

By the grace of the Goddess, Eunny's step didn't falter. She didn't skip like some giddy fool, either. No looking back. Forward only. Plenty of time for some lighthearted fun before any of the mess that came with labels and decisions.

She returned Gransen's look with a sly smile. "Oh, you know. Has he really not said anything?"

A long-suffering groan came in answer. "No, because he's a *gentleman.*" His lips quirked up. "Olly has been very chipper of late, though. Don't think I haven't noticed."

Eunny hummed innocently in response.

"Making Papa Granse proud." They stopped at a crossroads in the university's courtyard. "My two favorite people make a beautiful couple. I do good work."

"We aren't— Wait, what do you think *you* did?"

"Please. We both know—"

"We aren't a couple. It's not that serious, okay? We're *friends.*"

"No, Olly wouldn't just— He's way too far gone to see this as a friends-with-benefits thing. You do know that, right?" Gransen eyed her with something akin to reproach.

"Yeah, well, we haven't talked about it." A flush rose in her cheeks. "We're having fun. Can't ask for more than that."

Trunk came into view, a familiar, curly-haired head moving around just outside. Ollas looked up as the sound of their voices reached him.

"You could, if you wanted. Something holding you back?" A mischievous grin split Gransen's face. "Want me to ask? Olly might be embarrassed, but I have no shame."

"Get away from me." Eunny shoved him. In a louder voice, she called out, "Hey, Nev!"

Gransen laughed, waving to the two of them before wandering off toward the Grove.

Ollas faced her, pleasure lighting his face. "Eunny."

She stopped next to the wheelbarrow he'd parked alongside the now-empty patch that had held the delegation plants. A few carefully dug up plants lined the wheelbarrow's bed.

"What are you doing?" she asked.

"Zhen was right, we don't have much time left to work with these. Half the patch was already brown this morning. Propagating's not enough. If we don't figure out how to get them to flower and collect seed, they're gone."

Eunny held the door open so he could push the wheelbarrow inside. A row of the specialty terrarium boxes were arranged along the counter, already planted with cuttings from the delegation plants that had finished converting from grass to leaf. Over a dozen more that had shriveled and died filled a separate bin.

Eunny whistled. "You've been busy. Should've told me, Nev, I'd have come help."

"I know." He smiled at her. "I figured I'd see you in here soon enough."

Once the wheelbarrow was stowed next to the potting bench, Ollas went to her, hands reaching to skim her shoulders. "Is everything okay? I went by last night, but—"

She kissed him. "I'm fine. Went into town to see my aunt."

Relief filled his face, making a fresh spur of guilt poke at her insides. But no, that wasn't allowed. Not now, not at all. Only fun and light and nothing serious.

"Your mother is sweet. Promised to share all sorts of embarrassing stories about you," Eunny teased.

Ollas groaned. "Earthen take me, she would." His fingers

played with the ends of her hair. "Eunny, should we maybe talk about...this? Us."

Eunny stilled.

"Not— I don't mean anything bad." He huffed softly to himself and took her hand in his. "I mean...I'm in. For whatever this is. What you want. I'm here for whatever you'll give me."

Eunny felt her mouth drop open, but no response came to her lips. Emotions galloped through her head, the tenor changing with each blink of her eyes. Shock. Pleasure. A small amount of something cold that felt alarmingly like primordial fear. The way he laid himself out for her, the earnest way he held her gaze—on some level it both appealed to and terrified her. Unnerved her for a reason she couldn't comprehend.

A sliver of guilt was there, too. A hint of doubt that managed to pierce the other feelings.

"I'm here for all of it," he murmured. His eyes traveled over the trays of cuttings, then back to her face. "For everything we're going to do, it's...it's with you, and I'm happy."

He spoke so earnestly. From the heart, of a future, with hope and excitement that a part of her wanted to echo back to him. A rather large part. But that side of Eunny lived in ignorant bliss, too enamored with her forward-only view. It delighted in Ollas's declaration, content to be wrapped up in his words and think of them in simple, narrow terms. That side of her took his quiet words for *all of it* and *everything we're going to do* as glib. Pretended they weren't declarations from Ollas's mouth. But those were the kind of thoughts that led to the future and commitments. Planning, which implied Eunny making space for herself in his life. And him in hers. A form of permanence she didn't deserve, could only ruin if given an amount of time.

"What were you and Gransen talking about—?"

"Do we need to have labels?" she cut him off, keeping her tone playful. Before he could reply, she slid her hands across his chest. Let them drift lower, until they wrapped around his belt. "You're not in a rush, are you?"

"Not a rush, no, but it'd be—" His breath caught as she undid the buckle. "I, um, I was thinking…"

His voice dropped off along with his trousers. Eunny smirked up at him as she took his cock in her hand and slowly squeezed.

"I just thought—Oh, gods. Because we, we're—" Ollas groaned as she gave him a lazy pump back and forth. "Fuck. You're distracting *me*." His tone jumped as Eunny fondled his balls with her other hand.

"I should hope so," she said, smiling with teeth. Slowly, Eunny sank to her knees, pressing her cheek against his length. "I'm going to choke on this now, unless you wanted to keep talking?" She batted her eyelashes at him.

Ollas's eyes closed as he made a helpless sound and shook his head.

"Good boy. That's what I thought." Smugness colored her tone.

His cock bobbed in response, a bead of pre-come already glistening at the tip. Eunny kissed it, gaze drifting up until she met his eyes. "If it helps, yours is the only cock I'm interested in sucking."

She cut off his reply by taking him into her mouth and swallowing him down until her nose tickled his groin—like a slow inhale, steady, her tongue gliding along every hardened inch until his tip brushed the back of her throat. She resisted the urge to gag. Drew back with the same unhurried pace, sucking gently. His musk filled her nose, the salty earthiness of him spreading across her tongue.

Eunny paused at the tip, looking up at him again as she licked the head of his cock. Ollas was staring down at her, eyes almost glassy with lust.

"Just like I imagined," he murmured. "You are so…"

He groaned again as she took him deeper into her mouth, tongue circling the rim of his head, teasing at the ridge underneath. She kept going—long, slow slides up and down, increasing in pressure after each full stroke. His cock was impossibly hard, so thick she couldn't take him to the base anymore even as she tried to soften her throat for him. She took his balls into her hand again and gave them a squeeze, and a shiver ran through him. Made his hips jerk, the erratic movement sending him deeper into her mouth, enough to make her choke. She let it, throat closing, a short, sharp puff of air escaping through her nose as her lips firmed.

"Eunny, Eunny, I'm going to— Love, please." A hiss of breath escaped him as she hummed against the heat of him. "If you do that, I'll—" Ollas's babble ended in the most delectable moan as she took her time coming back to the surface.

"Nev," she murmured, pressing her lips against a raised vein on his cock, "it's hard to talk when my mouth is full."

Ollas was gripping the counter, a tremble running through his frame with the effort it took to hold himself back. Eunny reveled in it, felt a molten streak of desire run through her. Something hot and smug and possessive. To know that she did this to him. That he was hers, even if only for the moment.

His eyes finally opened, pupils blown wide as he stared down at her. "You are the most perfect, most beautiful…" He groaned as she lapped at his cockhead, pressing her tongue against the slit. "Most wicked."

Eunny smiled against his skin. "Says he of the greenhouse fetish," she teased. "This is what you've imagined, isn't it? Getting my knees dirty for you."

"It's…not quite like that." He hesitated, expression a mix of nervous and hopeful. No. Nervous and *hungry*. Enough to make Eunny press her thighs together.

"I'm listening."

"I have thought about it. Dreamed about it." He stroked her cheek with his knuckles. "What I'd do to you in here, if you'd let me."

She smirked, scrunching her nose. "Should I be worried?"

"Never." The word came out so low, fervent, and deep. "You'll enjoy it. I promise you that."

Eunny stood up, dusting herself off with exaggerated movements. "Bold words." She kept her tone light, playful. Gave no indication of how her heart sped up in her chest upon finding that perhaps she didn't have her sweet little bean all figured out just yet. She sauntered past him and put her hand on the door, turning the lock.

"Go on, then," she said, coming back to stand in front of him. She splayed her palms across his chest. "Surprise me."

The words had barely left her mouth before Ollas claimed it, one hand tilting her head up to him as his arm snaked around her waist to keep her close. An electric tingle ran across her skin with the gentle scrape of his short beard. He licked into her mouth, a rumble of pleasure sounding when she kissed him back. She smiled, tongue moving with purposeful strokes.

It only took a few steps for him to change their positions, moving her so that her ass bumped against the greenhouse's long countertop. His hands roamed over her body, pulled away her clothes enough to expose her more intimate parts. His thumbs slid beneath the band covering her breasts, pushed it up so he could gently tug at her nipples. She moaned, letting her fingers dig into his shoulders. He sucked her lower lip into his mouth, gave it a nibble, then pulled away, teeth flashing in a smile when she made a whine of protest.

Eunny shoved her panties down, kicking them out of the way. She dragged Ollas's hand down so he could feel how wet she was for him already. Desire coursed beneath her skin; her chest rose and fell with anticipatory breaths. "Color me surprised."

Ollas's cock bobbed up. Fully hard, thick as a godsdamned log. She reached for it, a pang of hunger vibrating deep in her core as her fingers wrapped around him. She reveled in how purpose-built he was. How he shuddered at her touch. It made a different form of hunger thrum beneath her skin. The air was charged, tingling around them.

He tapped the counter, a question in his eyes. "Yes?"

Eunny smirked, raising her leg with deliberate slowness until her knee nestled on one of the kneeling mats he so kindly moved into place. Ever a gentleman, even when indulging in his greenhouse kink. The thought made her swallow down a giggle as she folded her calf against the back of her thigh.

Ollas came up behind her, crowding in until his bulk pushed her forward, her belly going flat over the counter. He traced the line made by her elevated leg. "Still good?"

"What, have we done anything yet?" she teased, a daring lilt in her tone. "I know my limits, Nev. We're good until I say otherwise."

Ollas leaned over, his lips brushing her ear. "Bold words."

Eunny laughed—a mistake. Or not. Maybe it was more of an uncalculated yet perfect decision; it meant her mouth was open when he turned her head toward him and claimed her lips. Nothing sensual or lingering about it, only raw, with a hunger that matched her own. His cock slid against her folds, its length getting coated with her arousal as his mouth continued to slant over her again and again.

Just as his tip began to nose in, the thickness enough to make her squirm, Ollas froze.

"Fuck," he growled, pulling back. "I didn't bring a po—"

"I'll take one later." Eunny wiggled her hips. "Get back here."

Ollas looked torn, if only for a moment. A hoarse bark of a laugh escaped him when she grabbed his hand and made him palm the curve of her ass.

"You don't get to have me defiling school property and leave the job half done," she said.

His response was to snap his hips forward, burying himself to the hilt. Eunny cried out, jerking against the counter and his weight holding her fast. Her inner walls squeezed him, a sting of pain mixing with so much pleasure at the force. The way she had to stretch. She tried to hold on as he drew out and surged back in, once, twice...

Eunny went rigid as the orgasm stole over her, making her clench even tighter. A soft whimper punctuated her trembling as the climax bloomed over her, short yet intense. Ollas rode it out, balls-deep in her as his pelvis ground with slow, shallow thrusts.

As quickly as it had snuck up on her, the waves of ecstasy abated, and Eunny spiraled back down with a content sigh. Ollas's gentle ministrations ended. It caught her by surprise when he drove forward, enough that her raised leg shook. Yet he didn't slow. He placed his hands on either side of her waist, fingers holding her tight. Her breaths turned to pants, then cries, in sync with his thrusts. The friction had her back arching, a coil of need building at her center. One of his hands went to her bent, raised leg, shifting her open a scant bit more. Enough that she whimpered again when he thrust forward, bearing down.

Ollas's pace grew frenzied, more erratic, then he grunted, dropping over her back. His cock pulsed, heat spreading within as he emptied into her. He growled against the side of her neck, then finally went still. Eunny moaned softly, her pussy squeezing against his embedded length.

For a few moments, neither spoke, too busy catching their

respective breaths. Then Ollas pushed himself up enough to plant kisses along her upper back, nibbling at the top of her shoulder and her nape, all while remaining sheathed within her. His fingers trailed across her waist, slipping around to her front to rub a lazy circle around her clit. Zings of pleasure arced across her skin and made her shudder.

"Nev," she gasped out, clenching again as he pressed harder. How was he still so hard after coming? Little Nev, not just an animal but a beast.

"You have no idea," he said, voice low. "No idea how long I've wanted to do this."

He kissed her again, deeply, tongue stroking over hers. He swallowed down her whimper when he rolled her clit between his fingers. Kept working her over, winding her tighter and tighter with each tug. When her leg began to shake, she tried to slip it off the ledge, hands bracing against the wall for some kind of leverage. Ollas caught her behind the knee, pushing her back up. Held her wide, her pussy snug and filled by him. Made her hold the position as he bucked into her.

A nameless sense of need surged through her veins. It existed beyond her own body, rising to mesh with Ollas. There was a resonance between them, around them, building up and up until Eunny thought she might shatter. It made sparks dance beneath her skin, and behind closed eyes, her vision filled with golden light.

Ollas bent over her again as her hips began to stutter. "Come for me one more time, love."

She did, hard. Lost in the haze of passion and release, it felt as if her essence tangled with Ollas, exploding outward in a dusting of light. Of magic. But instead of fear, she knew only euphoria. If not for the weight of him holding her down, she'd have fallen off the counter with the violence of her spasms. As it was, the foot still touching the floor was useless, her leg buckling as he rutted into her. Another grunt spilled from his lips as his second climax peaked. Each of her contractions was mirrored by his cock throbbing, filling her with more of his seed. She'd be a mess when he finally pulled out.

Eh. What was one more type of fertilizer in the storage shed?

The thought made her snort with laughter even as satiation had her sagging across the counter.

"No," Ollas moaned, hips cuddled flush with her ass as he clung to her. "You're going to laugh me out."

The complaint only made her laugh harder. She nudged him. "You're squishing me."

Ollas dragged himself up, casting about until he found a stack of clean, folded towels on a nearby shelf. He offered her one, a nervous smile tugging at his lips. "Are you okay? I... That wasn't what I meant to do."

"No?" Eunny said, wiping herself off. "What happened to 'I've been dreaming about seducing you in the greenhouse, Eunny?'"

He blushed. "I think you seduced me first."

"Maybe. But I wasn't the one living out my fantasies." She stepped back into her trousers, then leaned against the counter. "So? Did reality disappoint?"

He indicated his still semi-hard cock. "Never."

Once they were both clothed, Eunny went to unlock the door. She turned back to see Ollas squinting around, blinking in confusion.

"What were we talking about before?" he asked, rubbing his eyes with his hands.

Perfect. Awkward conversations avoided for another day. Which should've done more to allay the tumult inside her when it came to this fun they were having and its inevitable expiration date. Because Eunny knew Ollas wouldn't say no to her. She'd exploit that goodness in him if need be.

"Can't help you there," she murmured, grabbing her cloak. "I've got to— Whoa! Nev, look!"

The fresh cuttings had exploded with new growth, leaves crowding against the glass. Ollas stared at them, fingertips pressed against the nearest enclosure. Abruptly, he pivoted away and dug out his journal, one hand scrabbling across the counter for a pencil.

Eunny found one hidden beneath an empty fertilizer bag and handed it over. "Have you ever seen—?"

"No, never," Ollas mumbled, frantically jotting down notes. He paused long enough to glance at her, an odd look on his face. Curious, yet apprehensive. "Did it feel like, just for a moment, um, like... magic?"

"No," Eunny said, the word coming out sharper than she meant.

A furrow marred his brow. His mouth opened, but uncertainty blocked any words.

Eunny forced herself to soften, an easy smile forming on her lips. "I know it was good, Nev, but let's not get carried away."

Ollas held her gaze. Something flickered behind his eyes, a moment of indecision, like he might argue. But then he relaxed, wiping a hand across his mouth and sighing. "Yeah, I guess you're right. It's just... unexpected."

"No argument from me." She took a step away. She had to get out of here, away, before he could dwell more on what had happened. Ask questions. "I need to check on something for the café."

He stopped her to give her a soft kiss before she could duck out the door. "See you later?"

"Sure," she said. "I'll find you."

Eunny stepped outside, heading back toward her apartment. A nervous shiver had her rubbing her hands briskly along her arms. It wasn't magic. She couldn't have just oozed light while Ollas was getting her off. If that was a thing, she'd have known about it by now, right?

Hard to argue with the evidence, though; something about those plants called to them. *Something* had taken advantage of how uninhibited they'd been in the moment. But pulling magic? No. Ollas didn't have a strong enough grasp of his own to have given the plants a hold, and Eunny, she hadn't summoned any of her light. This was just weird happenstance. She'd just had mind-blowing sex in a godsdamned greenhouse. Brought one of his fantasies to life. Shit, she'd certainly *felt* how enthusiastic he was about it. But plants and sex magic? Best to take her own advice and not get carried away.

"Pull it together, Song," she muttered.

Forward only. Nothing serious. If a small—infinitesimal, really—part of her was feeling some kind of way about discovering this kinky side of Ollas, it changed nothing. And that strange way he'd looked at her, the hesitancy in his voice when he'd asked if she'd felt any magic...

The way he'd been nervous to ask, but not necessarily surprised...

Eunny shook her head. She was slipping up around him in too many ways. Had been foolish enough to start to feel *safe*. It couldn't happen again.

Chapter Twenty

THOUGH THEIR INITIAL growth spurt had been impressive, in the days that followed, the secret delegation cuttings plateaued. The intangible pull from them was undeniable now, stronger and more pointed in its need. Whenever she was around the plants, Eunny felt a resonant tug at her center, at her inner sphere. It was a soundless whisper at her core, asking for her magic. In response, power hummed beneath her skin, just waiting to be let out. To be fed into the plants, laced through the living essence within them. It would've been simple, not so different a process to mixing healing remedies and giving the traces of magic in a leaf or a bud a gentle nudge. The mental motions came back to her with hardly any thought, so engrained were they from years of practice.

Eunny ignored the call. Easy; she'd spent six years learning how to keep such urges at bay. And though she didn't indulge Ollas and his greenhouse kink again, to prove an unspoken point between them, she kept the magical urge on a tight leash when they fucked at her place. It was easier now that she knew what to look for, now that she knew to ignore the spark that wanted to build. She didn't let it catch with Ollas's feather-light magic. Ignored the reflexive way her magic tried to carry over to the pair of water-rooted cuttings still on her table.

Much to Ollas's good-natured dismay.

He leaned down to peer at the jars, the plants unchanged despite the bedroom pursuits that had gone on around them. Huffing through his nose, Ollas pulled on his boots and muttered, "Can't blame me for trying."

Eunny hooked her arm around his neck and kissed him, scampering away when he tried to grab her waist. She fetched both of their cloaks from where they hung next to her front door. "I'll walk back with you. Granse wants to talk more about the café."

"You're going back to it?" Ollas asked.

She thought she heard in his voice a touch of the same regret she felt at the notion. "Not yet." A flutter of warmth spread through her at his visible relief. "I know he's ambitious, but it's still far from seaworthy. And it kind of should be, if a repair café is going to offer repairs, one would think."

They walked back toward the Grove, hoods pulled up against the evening's chill. Ollas kissed her goodbye before splitting off toward Trunk, intent on trying to infuse what he could of his earth magic into light-enhanced water for the delegation plants. Eunny watched his back disappear down the path, her cheeks puffing out in an aggrieved sigh. She'd have to sneak over later and see if applying her own magic after the fact would still work. A thought she didn't enjoy one bit, but needs must. Dae needed the plants. Rhell needed them. Eunny could just... deal with it. Give a scrap of her untrustworthy magic when Ollas was safely away, not a drop more than was strictly necessary. Then she'd be done and gone.

The thought of giving more of herself to the plants already left her feeling unsettled. But if she was alone, even if she lost control again, she couldn't hurt anyone. And no one would know. In the end, that was all that mattered.

Her knuckles had barely touched the wood of Gransen's door before he whipped it open and ushered her inside.

"Hello, boss." Gransen's eyes swept over her, a sly grin creeping across his face. "You look well. Flushed, I daresay. You haven't seen my erstwhile roomie, have you?"

"Shut up. It's cold outside." Eunny tossed her cloak over the back of a kitchen chair before taking a seat. Papers were strewn across the tabletop. "What's all this?" She spun a sheet around so she could read it. "Tea?"

Gransen shrugged, slouching into a chair across from her. "Just some ideas for a reopening celebration tea. Wanted something with excitement."

Eunny traced her finger along the scattered list of ingredients and effects. "Good luck finding fizzy hibiscus in bulk this time of year."

"Have any suggestions?" Gransen asked, rolling a pen beneath his finger.

She frowned in thought, then rattled off a few ideas, adding, "Ask Zhen for her source on purified goldleaf water. Steep with that at just below boiling and you'll get a nice, uplifting tea. Doesn't have the same mouthfeel, but it'll spark the feeling of joy you're after. Just limit how much people can drink. Get too buoyant and people start getting sloppy, you know? Plus, it's expensive. We're not rolling in gold."

Gransen had leaned forward, chin resting in his hands as he grinned at her.

"You're not writing any of this down," she said.

"Listen to you. Didn't even question that this was for the café. You're coming around on it. Love has changed you, boss."

Oh, Goddess break... "I'm not— No, it—"

"Eun, come on, you can admit it. You're doing apothecary

speak with basically no prompting. You're still here even though Olly's back on his feet."

"I have a commitment to the class, that's all," she protested. Her pulse ticked up, a dull roar starting to build in her ears.

"I've seen how you are with him. Warms my little heart to see two of my favorite people together."

"We're not," Eunny said, voice weakening. The roar grew louder. "It's not serious. It can't be."

The glee faded from Gransen's face. "Are you still on about the forgiveness thing?"

"The for— *Yes!*" Eunny cried, slamming her hands on the table as she stood. "I'm not in love with Ollas. I'm *atoning*. I always will be. Why is that so hard for you to understand?"

Gransen stared at her, eyes wide with shock.

Her breath came sharp and fast, something like panic rising in her chest. She was so stupid. Thinking she could traipse around here, keep her guard up. She'd never thought she'd weaken, forget she couldn't have this life. Didn't *deserve* it. But it had been too easy to settle in at the Grove, on campus. An off-hand comment about herbalism, correcting wayward Ennis, she'd thought it was nothing. She'd never realized how slowly she'd come to be at ease. How she'd reached out and grabbed hold of some semblance of what her life might've been. Doing apothecary work for the school. Using her skills to aid the fight against the poison in Rhell. Calling on her magic. She'd done all those things, and somewhere along the way, she'd lost her vigilance. Been lulled into feeling *safe*.

Somewhere along the way, Eunny had stopped looking at Ollas and feeling guilt.

"Maybe at first," Gransen said slowly, warily, as if he was afraid she would explode. "But I've seen the way you two are together. I know you, both of you. You're— You're *good*. Right."

Eunny shook her head, denial turning her stomach.

"I look at how you two are and...I want that. Someday," Gransen murmured, with rare solemnity. "I know this started out of guilt, but you're really telling me you haven't developed some feelings?"

Yes, and what a mistake that had been. Weakness on her part, and maybe even cruelty, because she was never going to stay. Couldn't.

"No," she said, quiet but steady. "I can't."

"He doesn't blame—"

"I do." She looked down at her hands. "When I see him... Until I can do that and not remember how it felt to have my magic tear him apart, there's no forgiveness. I won't believe in it."

Gransen's mouth opened, but then he just sighed, wilting in defeat.

A soft, hesitant throat-clearing broke through the heavy silence, drawing Eunny and Gransen's attention to the door. The open door, Ollas framed within it, a flurry of emotion on his face. Shock, and hurt, yet that was too simple a word for what Eunny saw when their eyes met.

"Ollas." Her voice came out as a whisper. No need to ask how much he'd heard. What did it matter, really, when he'd clearly heard the end?

His expression didn't quite shutter—Ollas wasn't capable of that—but she watched him push his disappointment away as he gathered himself to speak. "There's been a break-in at Trunk."

"What?" Eunny and Gransen said at once.

Ollas turned away, his arm stiff as he gestured for them to follow. "The delegation plants. They're all gone."

Chapter Twenty-One

GRANSEN OPTED TO STAY BEHIND, not being involved in their project. Silence loomed heavy and awkward between Ollas and Eunny as they rushed down to the storage greenhouse. Ollas hated it but didn't trust himself to break it, not yet. Not when his thoughts were still twisted up in Eunny's words. How she'd yelled at Gransen, been so adamant in her denials. Her honesty, no less brutal for its truthfulness. Perhaps it was good for him to hear it, this affirmation that when Eunny looked at him, she couldn't see past the specter of guilt. Then again, weren't they the same in that? Only, Eunny still didn't know the whole truth. Couldn't, not if she didn't remember the specifics of that day. The details surrounding the moment her magic had gone so wrong. The cause. He'd have to tell her, make her listen instead of letting her wave away his feeble attempts. He'd have to stop being a coward.

But not yet. There were more pressing matters at hand. He cast a quick glance her way and found anxiety mirrored in Eunny's face before she broke eye contact. The emotions were too raw. Given the crime scene in the greenhouse, stress levels would only get worse over the course of the night.

Professor Rai and Zhenya were already in Trunk, their expressions grim when the others approached.

"I've alerted Castle," Rai said, naming the manager of the greenhouse complex. "No one else knows, and I would like it kept that way. I'll inform the dean."

Ollas nodded in acknowledgement. A dull form of numbness crept over him as he stared around the rear antechamber. The floor was a mess of tipped over glass jars and spilled substrate. Only one of the jars had broken, but each was empty; not even a broken-off leaf remained of the delegation plants. The bucket of scraps for the compost piles had been emptied. The rest of the rack where the jars had been was eerily clean and ordinary compared to the disarray on the ground. As if the thief had known exactly what to take. Which made no sense. There were valuable specimens in Trunk. Not in the tidiest of shape, or ones that would fetch the highest prices compared to what the grovetenders kept elsewhere, but still more valuable than the anonymous plants that had been growing outside for the last six years. Though Ollas had a gut feeling they were special, he had no proof. Neither Zhenya nor Rai had detected anything unique or magical about them, and if grovetenders of their caliber could not, then why would anyone else?

"I was coming in to test some different amendments," Ollas said in a dull tone. "No one was in here. I didn't pass anyone on the way in."

Not that he'd been looking especially hard. It was the greenhouse complex; students and staff came and went all the time. The later hour was of no consequence, either, since a full moon approached and Magisters' experiments were being readied for it.

As far as finding Trunk undisturbed—except for the rear antechamber—that wasn't so surprising, either. It was Trunk, the storage greenhouse. While the doors technically locked—as demonstrated by his escapades with Eunny—no one had bothered with locking Trunk for security reasons in years. There was no need amongst the student body, and besides, it was Sylveren. Ollas wasn't naïve enough to say sabotage never happened on campus, but a theft like this?

"You're certain no one else knows about your private work?" Rai said.

Ollas felt Eunny glance at him as he shook his head. "I can't be certain of who all might've seen it, but everyone I've talked to about it in depth is here."

"I haven't heard anyone mention them either," Zhenya added.

Rai frowned, one long finger tapping against his crossed arms as he thought. "We'll need to return to keeping the buildings locked at all times. You have your keys?" He gave Ollas and Zhenya questioning looks.

They both nodded.

"Good. I doubt the thieves will return, seeing as they came with single-minded purpose, but we should all be on alert just in case." Rai shook his head, nostrils flaring with his frustrated sigh. "I'll speak to the dean about getting the Sentinels involved."

Rai and Zhenya left in search of the dean and greenhouse manager respectively. Ollas moved to grab a broom, but Eunny's hand on his arm stopped him.

"Ollas," she said, hesitance in her voice and in the way she slowly raised her eyes to him. "What I said... What you heard, I—"

He'd been a fool to think their comfort with one another was indicative of something more. That she could ever want it. That she could ever fall in love with someone like him. Only lust. But hadn't he said he was in for whatever she'd give him? Seeing the shame on her face, the guilt that he'd wanted so badly to erase... Ollas had never wanted to be the cause for it. Not again, anyway.

He couldn't take back his foolish choice all those years ago, letting his selfish desire to feel her healing magic override the signs of her exhaustion. Eunny had made it clear that he couldn't change her mind over her long-held guilt.

But he could do something now, and keep the past from repeating.

Ollas took her face between his hands, leaning down so his forehead pressed against hers as he murmured, "We agreed on no labels, right?" He gave her a shaky smile. "No spoiling the fun. And I think we could use some of that right now."

Eunny sagged with such visible relief that Ollas wondered if she could hear how those words broke him inside.

It was after midnight by the time Eunny finally stumbled back to her apartment. She collapsed on her bed, too tired to undress. They'd cleaned up the mess of the greenhouse and produced a few theories on who would want to steal the plants. Or who would even know about them. Ollas had his Sentinels contacts to ask, but it made no sense why any of them would invade Trunk.

Eunny rolled onto her back and stared up at the ceiling. Tried not to think about how hollow Ollas had been with her. The forced casualness as they'd worked. Not his shy, sweet awkwardness like when they'd first been getting used to each other. No comfortable, familiar silence.

It shouldn't have bothered her so much. Now he knew how she felt. What her limits were. They were on the same page about the seriousness, or lack thereof, of their casual fun.

Except... it hurt. She had hurt him. Couldn't pretend that

she hadn't noticed his attraction. She'd enjoyed it. Him. Even if she'd never meant to let any such feelings get that far. Eunny had tried so hard to avoid getting into this mess.

Did you, though? a traitorous voice asked. All her teasing, flirting with Ollas to see him flush. Could she really say, from the moment she'd indulged in that kiss, that she'd been trying to avoid something real? That sleeping with Ollas had been simple, casual sex? That she hadn't loved being called his goddess, hadn't cared about the sentiments precisely because they came from him?

And beyond the carnal, she hadn't exactly clung to her convictions of distance. Eunny felt... not quite at home in the Grove, but something closer to peace than she'd ever felt with Song's Scrap. She could finally brush her fingers along the edge of her old apothecary work. Feel a touch of joy again instead of revulsion and anger and guilt. No, in the end, she hadn't tried so hard to keep her distance. Agreeing to stay on for the elective, to help with those damned weeds. Feeling the spark, as Dae had said. Feeling comfortable enough with Ollas that the beliefs she'd held for so long, couched in fear and doubt, started to soften—only a little, but they had. She had. With him, Eunny had let her mind start to change.

She exhaled slowly, emotions mixing with exhaustion as her mind tried to wrap itself around these revelations and what they meant. What she should do. The tumult was such that it took a moment for her to recognize a tug at the edge of her mind. A hum in the air, beneath her skin, homing in on her center. The steady pulse of not her heartbeat but something else. A different thrum of life, insistent, and so familiar when she paid attention.

Eunny sat up, looking at her kitchen counter and the two cuttings she had floating in water.

Eunny huddled outside of Trunk, unable to gain entrance since she wasn't staff, and waited for Ollas to arrive. The cuttings were tucked into her cloak's inner pockets, each snug in a fist-sized jar, roots happily submerged in a watery gel she'd infused with her magic. The plants exuded a buzzy energy palpable through the thin glass of their containers, as if it could hardly be contained in their, well, skin, or whatever the plant equivalent was.

She rested her head against the greenhouse door, eyes closing. Sleep had been more illusion than reality. She'd spent hours reviewing old apothecary notes against the meager knowledge she'd gained thus far in helping with the elective, and nervousness at reaching for her magic again didn't amount to much rest. Using her magic of her own volition. Revealing it. Because after tonight, Eunny didn't know how she'd be able to keep its existence a secret any longer. The pair of cuttings had responded well to her magic, their innate call building even more. Linking her to them, them to her.

And to Ollas. The more she let herself feel the plants' resonance—stopped resisting it and truly listened—other familiarities arose. The restlessness and intangible pull that had been growing since the summer. Little notes in the magic that she knew instinctively were Ollas. Traces of his magic embedded in the plants like nuggets of gold. They were unmistakable now that she knew to look. If she could feel the pieces of him in the spell that bound them, then he should be able to find the elements of her.

The plants had put out even more of their glossy green leaves. Eunny was no gardener, but to her novice eye, they looked close to flowering. If she could nudge one to bloom, just one, so they could collect the seeds, that was all she needed.

Seeds would buy them time to figure out what the plants even *were* that would incite theft. Or, buy *someone* the time needed; Eunny wasn't opposed to taking Zhenya's advice and passing the whole mess off to someone else. Presuming the imprinting process had only been spelled into the initial batch of seeds. But she'd deal with that if it came up.

"Eunny?"

She startled. "Shit! Scared the life out of me, Nev."

"Sorry," Ollas murmured. He inclined his head toward the door. "You wanted to meet?"

"I'll tell you inside."

Ollas let them into the greenhouse. Eunny checked the antechambers, confirming they were empty before re-locking the main entrance. Ollas watched her, brows knitting together in confusion, but didn't speak. She steeled herself, sucking in a deep breath before opening the fronts of her cloak.

"We're not out of this yet." She revealed the two glass jars she carried. "I think they're about to flower."

His eyes widened, mouth dropping open. As recognition hit, he nodded slowly, attention more on her than the cuttings. He lifted his hand, calling a few quavery yellow-white sparks. "I'm feeling pretty good today. Want to see if we can push them to bloom?"

Her mental preparation for the moment wavered. "I-I... Ollas, I can't—"

"Eunny." Her name was spoken with such calm, at odds with her frenetic babble. Ollas reached past her to activate the opacity charm enchanted onto the greenhouse's glass windows. Meant to shield the greenhouse from rare days of intense summer sun, the enchantment blurred them so they resembled indistinct silhouettes to outside view.

"The spell needs both of us." Ollas grabbed a deep planting tray, put a scoop of corrupted earth into the bottom, and set the tray between them on the counter. He held her gaze. "I can try first, see if I can wake them."

They were standing beside each other again, close enough that Eunny could feel the warmth emanating from his skin. One small movement of her elbow and she'd touch him. And yet. They were so close, but there might as well have been an ocean between them. Vast and ever so empty. Devoid of anything so solid as words. Words that he'd implied with his careful phrasing and knowing—maybe even *encouraging*—looks. Words that she refused to say. Once they became sounds, concrete things uttered from her mouth, there was no taking them back. Speaking was admitting.

But the way Ollas looked at her, his thready magic flickering in his palm, the lack of surprise in his tone when he spoke... He knew. But he wouldn't force her to admit it aloud. Instead, he'd let her show him without words.

At her tiny nod, Ollas took one of the cuttings and gently buried the stem. Then he sank his fingers into the dirt until his palm rested on the surface. Eunny's hand jumped up—whether to stop him or something else, she didn't know. She forgot to breathe, eyes glued to where his hand disappeared into the poisoned ground.

A faint, unsteady glow built around Ollas's palm. His magic, weak and thready like a guttering candle but still present.

She held herself still, swallowed back her nerves as a new presence cropped up in her mind. A familiar tug at her magic. Only, this time, it felt so much more alive.

The cutting still enclosed in its jar buzzed softly against the glass, while its twin fluttered against Ollas's hand.

Their seeds, their *plants*, called to her. Or rather, the kernel of magic she'd unwittingly left behind in them did. An inherent pull that grew to a steady pulse, reverberating in her head.

An itch built at Eunny's fingertips, magic pooling in her

palms, just beneath the skin. It came to her without conscious thought. Like second nature, as it once had. Maybe it always would—did, *had*—if she had ever let herself notice.

Moving slowly and hesitantly, Eunny placed her hand beside Ollas's, letting her pinky brush his. He stared at her, a sense of wonder morphing into delight. Happiness. Maybe even pride? Her trust hadn't gone unnoticed, but then of course it wouldn't. This was Ollas, and he was too good.

She couldn't think about that. His magic had been enough to awaken the plants, to encourage tiny nubbins to form amongst the leaves, but it hadn't carried them all the way. Maybe his magic was too weak. Or maybe they'd always needed something else. The touch of both the people who'd imprinted on them. The buds woke and hungered for the energy to be whole.

A rushing sensation coursed through Eunny's mind. An understanding that a process had started that couldn't be paused, only fueled or killed.

Eyes closing, Eunny let a trickle of her magic go. Let it spread into the soil a few droplets at a time. Felt the roots wick it up, her magic winding around the blinking rise and fall of Ollas's own.

The tiny buds reacted with blazing speed, blooms swelling until they seemed to burst. Petals fanned out in Eunny's mind's eye; the shape of the plants formed in her head, lit up with her magic.

Beside her, Ollas tensed with concentration as he called for more of his own power.

But he wasn't much above a mundane, bless him, his essence low and already down to the dregs with his efforts. The flowers stretched outward, hungry for more magic, shaking when they came up nearly dry.

Eunny's magic responded. Through it, she felt the plants'

need for her light, thanks to those drops of magic fed so long ago when they were mere seeds. Her magic remembered, like drawn to like, eager to feed the dearth until all were equal. Easily done. All it required was magic, and hers had never left. Only been buried. Repressed for so long that there were little things she'd forgotten.

Nothing like recurrence to jog the memory.

Instead of a few drops of magic carefully meted out by her command, Eunny's magic surged. Was *pulled* from her, rushing out into the dirt, watering the plant with her light. Her eyes opened. The cutting had exploded with small blossoms, their petals a stark crimson against the deep green of the foliage. They waved in the torrent of her magic, pinpoint sparks floating up and dissipating with an almost inaudible hiss.

Little bursts of gold, so reminiscent of popping bubbles.

When one landed on her skin, the minute crackle made her jump. It was different… yet so horribly familiar. The way her magic poured out of her, the rushing, slipping feeling, it turned her mouth sour. Panic rose in her throat as she remembered the last time her magic had surged like this.

Eunny flung herself away, wrenching on her magic. It resisted, her threads of golden-white light tangling with Ollas's strands. His weaker magic called for more of hers, for help.

"No!" She slammed down on the connection, on the subtle warmth in her chest. Ripped herself free of their snarled mess of lines. Didn't think of the consequences, her mind grasping on to a single imperative: *away*. Only banging into the rack of plants across the aisle stopped her from going further.

Ollas's hand jerked as if he'd been stung. He turned to her, concern etched across his face at seeing her collapsed against the opposite rack.

"Eunny?" He reached out to comfort her.

"Don't," she bit out, flinching away. "Just— Oh, gods. Ollas!"

His skin, on the hand that had been in the dirt, the one that had touched her magic, was now an angry, inflamed red.

Icy fear washed over her. "Ollas, did I…?" she moaned.

He glanced down at his hand, blinking rapidly. His expression cleared. "No, Eunny, you didn't do this. It's from the blight. It'll clear in a moment. This wasn't you, see?"

Eunny shrank from his proffered hand, the metal edge of the shelf digging into her back. She didn't want to see. Didn't want to feel or know or—

"Eunny, you didn't lose control." He spoke softly to her, as if soothing a wild animal. "Your magic is fine."

She shook her head. Refused to understand his meaning. To believe. "No. It happened again, Ollas." A humorless laugh fell from her mouth. "I'm the Healer Who Hurts. I can never take that back. I hurt you *again*."

"You didn't—"

"You knew I still had it," she whispered.

"You used it around me. It's not much, but I do have some magic, remember?" he said, keeping his tone light as if attempting to ease the wall of tension rising between them. "I wanted to bring it up, I just didn't know how. I thought if you were comfortable with me, eventually you'd tell me on your own."

"I don't want to be comfortable with it, Ollas! I don't want to use it. I hate it."

"Why?" he asked. He looked so lost, pleading with her for guidance.

She slashed her arm through the air in the direction of the delegation plant cutting. It had shriveled under the volatile push and pull of magic, every bloom now browned and fallen to the bottom of the tray.

"Because it failed me. I hurt you, and when I use it, I remember..." Eunny shook her head violently. "I remember that day. That fucking moment. I have to relive the feeling of you breaking apart beneath my godsdamned fingers every time I use it. I don't know how you can stand there and not hate me."

Ollas reached for her again, desperation in every motion, replaced by anguish when she leaned away. "I could never hate you. I don't blame you, not for any of it."

Eunny's eyes burned with the threat of tears. She blinked them away, shoulders slumping as she gazed at him. No matter what she did, she ended up hurting him, and Ollas was so good, he still tried to take the blame. Make her happy. Because he was all in, as he'd said. He would never give up. Not of his own volition.

"You heard what I said to Gransen. I hurt you, Ollas. I haven't forgiven myself for it. I don't know that I ever will." She pressed her palms against her face. "I fucked up in letting us— It was a mistake—"

"It was my fault, Eunny."

"What? No, it wasn't."

"I need you to remember," he said, an earnest look back on his face.

Eunny stared at him.

"I need you to remember my part in it." His voice went quiet. Somber. "I need you to remember, and love me anyway."

"*Love* you?" Eunny's voice cracked.

"Yes," Ollas said, and when he smiled at her, it held such sadness it could almost pierce the cloud of fear and remorse swirling around her. "If you can. If you ever could."

Eunny raked a hand through her hair. "It's not you— I mean, it is, but it's not that I could never care about you as a person—"

"I'd always hoped so," he murmured. "But, maybe we can't believe the best in each other. Not until we know the worst."

"What are you talking about? Ollas, you're the best person—"

"It's my fault you lost control of your magic," he said, an edge to his tone. "Having the seeds on me, letting you heal me even though—"

"I'm the one who insisted!"

"I touched your magic, Eunny. I wanted to know what you felt like," he whispered. "Just once. Because I knew you'd never look at me twice. Not like that."

Eunny glared at him, hand slicing through the air as she indicated the two of them. "So much for that theory, you dipshit." Frustration had her grinding her teeth. "You aren't safe around me—"

"I love you. I've been in love with you forever," Ollas said, voice soft, imploring. "It kills me that you are still in pain because of what *I* did. If you can't believe my words, then I need you to *remember* what I did."

Eunny didn't realize that she'd been inching away, her head shaking in vague denial, until she bumped against the antechamber's door. She yanked it open and fled.

Ollas made no sound to stop her.

"Get over here, Nev."

Ollas complied, trying to hide the tremble in his limbs. He hoped Eunny would attribute it to his injuries rather than the mix of nerves and giddiness at her nearness coursing through him. Though pain erupted from a dozen points along his body, the moment she laid a glowing golden hand on him, everything began to recede. Like kneading a knotted muscle, her magic seeped into the wound on his arm and pressed, relieving some of the fire.

Yet, Eunny's magic wavered. It was not sparse or ribbony like Ollas's own pitiful gift, which had never been strong or plentiful, but weakened with exhaustion. While she could take some of the sting out of his arm, the wound itself remained unchanged, her magic lingering just below the surface of his skin.

"Eunny," he murmured.

She was muttering to herself, eyes closed, dark hair plastered to her cheeks from the heavy rain. Her light brown skin was ashen, weariness stealing the energy he was so used to seeing in her face. Her fingers shook as they tensed around his forearm.

He hated to see her in such a state. Knew she'd been stretching herself thin trying to patch everyone up. He should've refused when she'd beckoned him over. But he hadn't, and years of knowing one another meant he knew she'd be too stubborn to admit defeat now. She needed help, but the Coalition's delegation hadn't seen fit to bring a mender along who specialized in direct healings. There wasn't even another light mage who could act as a power source.

Ollas blinked, mind skipping along that train of thought. All magic had been derived from the Goddess Syvrine's light, or so the legends said, before breaking off to the various specialties. In his grovetending, sometimes Ollas, with a nudge from his own weak magic, had been able to get an enchantment to take hold by bridging the arcane essence inherent in a plant with that of the spellwork. Normally, a mender of Eunny's skill wouldn't need his assistance, even though her specialization lay in mixing healing blends and remedies, but tired as she was now? Surely, any help he could give wouldn't go amiss. And... he would get to feel her magic. The shape of it. Would know the taste of Eunny's light as it intertwined with his, if only just for a moment. He'd likely never get such a chance again.

"Eunny," Ollas mumbled.

"What, Nev? I'm trying to think here," she muttered back. Her jaw tensed as she struggled to channel more of her light.

"Let me help." Timidly, Ollas placed his free hand on top of hers just enough for the tips of their fingers to overlap. "I can try to guide you..."

Ollas reached for his light, managing to draw up a few flickering dots. He felt Eunny's magic respond, a line rising to wrap around his little sparks. It drew more, created a strange binding as Eunny's magic sank back into his flesh.

The wound on his arm went numb. Then cold, so cold it throbbed. His arm lay folded over his chest, and beneath it, dozens of spots of heat lit up. They seared through the fabric of his shirt and cloak, enveloping his skin. Fire spread across his wound, turning the icy pain to a burn. It felt like a hundred tiny brands against his skin, concentrated around one spot on his chest—

The seed packet he'd been examining in the tent. The one he'd carelessly stuck in his pocket before racing out to answer the horn calls.

It made no sense; they hadn't registered as anything magical when he'd reached out. But now, something had woken. Was wrapping like a fist around his magic, dragging erratic, weak sparks from his inner sphere that tangled with the lines of Eunny's magic.

She fought back. Ollas couldn't explain it, but he felt her resist the invisible hand pulling the snarl of their magic out.

She lost the battle. Her mental grip weakened, and a blaze of arcane heat flashed across Ollas's body. Every muscle seized, a scream lodging in his throat. When darkness finally claimed him, it was a blessing.

Chapter Twenty-Two

Coming back to Sylveren had been a mistake. Eunny had known it would be, but she'd done it anyway. Gave in for the creature comforts of a short walk and a chance to live in the Grove. To feel like she belonged. She'd escaped the everyday drudgery of slogging through her café full of junk, but in doing so had let herself forget that she'd surrounded herself with the mundane for a reason. She had thrown caution aside despite her better judgment. Been tempted by Ollas with his shy, earnest awkwardness. Let herself be charmed. She'd chased after the notion of some spark they might have together and convinced herself it would be okay if it wasn't meant to last.

Eunny blew past the university's outer gate and stomped toward town. It was raining again, harder this time than the mist that had pervaded the Valley the last few days. The rain had been the start of all of this. If the weather had been fairer, Song's Scrap wouldn't have collapsed. Ollas wouldn't have been hurt. She wouldn't have gone begging him to let her *help*, and she'd never have fallen in that godsdamned patch of grass, would never have accidentally fed it some of her magic and triggered the fucking imprinting spell and gotten sucked into this. Fucking. Mess.

Still, the rain gave her an excuse to huddle in the depths of her cloak and refuse eye contact with the few travelers she passed, and she welcomed it.

A part of her knew that she was being irrational. That she was scared, and had been for a long time. It'd been nice to let some of that fear go, if only for a little while. But she couldn't afford such lapses. Fear was like pain, meant to be felt for a reason. Ignoring put not only her at peril but Ollas, too. Maybe the burn on his hand had come from the dirt, as he'd said. Or maybe it was because of her. Because she'd lost control, or because she'd panicked. Either way, Eunny was the cause. His denial was nothing more than another kind-hearted attempt to protect her.

It was my fault, he'd said. *I touched your magic.*

Because he'd wanted to feel it, that part of her. He thought that featherlight pluck of his magic had been the catalyst for her disastrous meltdown. His earnest shame was almost cute, except Eunny couldn't feel further from laughing. He of such little magic, not realizing how collaboration and joining like that was fairly standard. When she finally let herself think back on that awful day, to remember his part in it as he'd begged her to do, she picked up on those minute flutters. Recognized the signature of his magic and how it felt, realized how many times she'd been experiencing flickers of it throughout their fling. Oh, Ollas, thinking he'd been to blame all these years, too. No, that was all hers.

He deserved better. Someone whose first response wasn't flight at his declaration of... love. Could he really? *Her?* How could he even know?

It didn't matter. Ollas might think he was *in* for whatever mess she entailed, but Eunny was not. Ollas—sweet, caring

Nev—he deserved someone who gave him honesty back. Eunny ran. He'd chosen her and all his confession did was fill her with an unnamable fear. It was just...wrong. He couldn't, shouldn't, feel like that about her. The Homegrown Hero couldn't be in love with the Healer Who Hurts. The woman who would rather hide than have anything to do with magic, even if it meant keeping herself from the work that was her calling.

Mending wasn't absolute, wasn't perfect or without risks; Eunny knew that. It couldn't fix all ills. Magic worked until it didn't, as the saying went. She wasn't the first to have an accident. Wouldn't be the last, either. Eunny understood the logic, the reality, but she couldn't find comfort in it. Ollas's forgiveness should've been freeing, yet she couldn't convince herself to believe. Whenever a shred of hope, of longing for the kind of life she might have if she put faith in him, rose, guilt was never far away.

This thing with Ollas had been a mistake. He had weakened her resolve, left her vulnerable to the myriad temptations of magic and belonging that were everywhere in the Valley. She'd cut herself off from the magic community before. She could do it again.

Eunny stopped outside the damaged building. Her repair café. Gransen had worked faster than she'd imagined; it looked under construction rather than coming back from collapse. She moved to unlock the front door, then shook her head, ambling around the side to peer in at the darkened main room. Still a mess inside, but an organized one. Ready for her to start again. Go back to the way things were, with her in town and only indirect contact with the school. With Ollas. She could go back to a few words of small talk.

She could move on and forget. She knew such apathy was in her; she'd done it before. Could pare every tender piece away until she was stone again. Nothing but superficial pleasantries on the outside, allowing no one in. But it would be harder this time.

Movement, a reflection in the glass of the café's rear window, caught Eunny's eye. A temporary ladder had replaced the broken stairway outside of the living quarters over the tearoom. Eunny turned in time to see a black cloak disappear inside the loft.

Eunny scampered after as quietly as she could, mouthing a prayer to the Goddess that the ladder wouldn't creak. Or break beneath her. Peering over the top rung, Eunny watched as her mother prowled around the small loft. She held a small light globe in one hand and a scrap of paper in the other, consulting it on occasion while picking through Eunny's old stash of tea and other blending ingredients.

"What are you doing?" Eunny snapped, pulling herself up the rest of the way so she could follow her mother into the loft.

Bioon startled, hand dropping to her cloak's pocket as she doused the light globe. Her arm tensed, and Eunny had a brief, intense moment of awe as the prospect of her mother pulling a weapon on her flitted through her mind. But then Bioon's stance eased as recognition crossed her face. "Eunji."

"Mother." Eunny stalked forward. "Why are you sneaking around my house? Does Auntie Yerina—"

"Your house? Don't be ridiculous. This hovel is hardly livable." Bioon gave the torn-up floor and gaping hole near the front a disdainful look. "You clearly haven't been staying here."

"I've been at the school. Again, what are you—" Eunny darted forward and snatched at the paper in her mother's hand, managing to tear half free. She stared at the hastily sketched lines depicting the delegation plant. "What the fuck is this?"

"Keep your voice down," Bioon said mildly. "You don't want to attract attention."

"I think I do." Eunny brandished the scrap of paper. "It was you! The fucking Coalition, I should've guessed. I can't believe you broke into a Sylveren building. The Sentinels—"

"If you force my hand, Eunji, the Sentinels or any other security you call will find remnants of your precious plants being smuggled out in Mighty Leaf packaging, courtesy of my sister."

Eunny stared at her mother. "What?"

Bioon's smile was pitying. "You know, Yeri would probably admit to it, if she thought it would help me."

"You— She isn't even involved in this!" Eunny hissed. "You'd go down, too."

"My employers would take care of me." Bioon's tone cooled. "My sister would not be so fortunate. Or do you want to take that chance?"

A part of her wanted to call her mother's bluff, but Eunny thought of Yerina, so desperate for any semblance of familial affection between them. How she continued to write to her sister, dismissing Bioon's constant snubs and always offering up her heart. Maybe they could prove Yerina's innocence, but not before it caused problems for the Mighty Leaf. Bioon would sully the tearoom's name, interfere with trade contracts, and that was presuming Yerina wasn't hauled down to Central for any legal proceedings. Not to mention the damage it would cause between the sisters. For one short, savage moment, Eunny considered it, wondering if such a betrayal would finally make her aunt see the truth.

She couldn't do it.

"Why do you even want them? The plants are fucking dying anyway. What good are they to you?"

Bioon said nothing.

"They're from the delegation. I remember the seeds. What is the Coalition doing—"

"I did warn you not to meddle in Coalition affairs," Bioon

murmured. "You should've known to leave well enough alone. The Coalition is very protective of its property."

"They don't belong to you," Eunny snarled. "They were part of the Eyllic deal, right? Isn't that why you had me test them? And since the delegation went to shit, I imagine the Sentinels would dispute your claims."

"They're welcome to try."

The mocking smile on her mother's lips made Eunny want to scream. Or slap it from her face. It filled her with such rage that her hands shook as she fisted them at her sides. "I won't let you get away with this."

"Oh?"

Eunny summoned a mocking smile of her own. "You missed a spot." Maybe. She couldn't remember what had happened to the sole remaining cutting after she'd fled from Trunk. But Bioon didn't know that. She thought her Coalition goons had already cleared out the place. "Return the plants, or I'll—"

"Turn them over to me willingly, and this all goes away," Bioon said, tone cold but unwavering. "Force my hand and it will go badly."

"Just try it. You might've been able to sneak into the most unused greenhouse, but let's see the might of the Coalition try and invade Sylveren University," Eunny taunted.

"Don't be ridiculous. The Coalition owns everything from the delegation, including goods brought by the Eyllics. They will get them, Eunji. They can assert the Law of Eminence and get the Lower Council to order your surrendering possession if they must, and the university will comply. Relinquish your plants without fuss"—Bioon gave her a contemptuous look— "or they will be taken from you, and you can say goodbye to Yeri and her pathetic tea shop."

"You hateful bitch."

Bioon stared at her in silence for a long moment. Her eyes

pressed closed, nostrils flaring as she inhaled, shoulders tensing.

Eunny fought to keep herself still. Would this be the time her mother finally yelled back? They'd fought all Eunny's life, but Bioon cut with scorn, not volume. Eunny was the one who yelled and screamed. Tantrums were beneath her mother. Or perhaps one needed to care more, to *feel* more, to have those kinds of feelings and fights. Doubtless, her mother had been called worse by people whose opinions actually mattered to her.

Bioon tossed her ripped half of the plant drawing aside as she swept toward the loft's door. "I've given you your options. My colleagues will be on the next windrunner up here. Make your choice or one will be made for you."

Eunny wasn't sure how long she stood staring at the blank space where her mother had been. With numb fingers, she retrieved the paper, crumpling it into a ball before stuffing it in her pocket. She slowly followed the same trail Bioon had taken, hesitating outside the Mighty Leaf's back door. The warmth and sounds of merriment were too much for her mood right now.

A form paused beyond the door's window, then Auntie Yerina appeared in the doorway. "Eunny! I didn't know you were here. Your mother just—"

Eunny didn't know what her face looked like, but it couldn't have been good. Yerina hurried forward, arms wrapping around her shoulders.

"Eunny. I'm sorry. Whatever it was, give her time. She'll come around and—"

Same old Yerina, coming to her hateful little sister's defense. Not even questioning what Bioon had done, or how Bioon contributed to the perennial fights and acrimony always brewing between mother and daughter. No, Yerina was always playing peacemaker, endeavoring for Eunny to be better, more understanding. Never a word spoken against Bioon, *ever*. Yerina made such an easy target that it was no wonder Bioon took advantage. Bioon was probably right in thinking that Yerina would shoulder the blame, too; anything for her precious sister, no matter how undeserving she was. And Eunny passively went along, Bioon pulling her strings, too.

Eunny shrugged out of her aunt's embrace. "Are you serious? She's always been like this. She's a fucking bitch who—"

"She's your mother, Eunny," Yerina said in a pained voice. "I know she can be cold. I know that, but she'll—"

"Why do you defend her? Why do you even try with her?" Eunny yelled. "She hates you. You do know that, right? She hates you and just uses you whenever she wants something. She uses everybody, and we're all just too stupid to do anything about it."

Blinking back angry tears, Eunny dashed out of the room.

Chapter Twenty-Three

LIFE HAD SEEN fit to give Ollas a second chance, and he'd royally fucked it up. Eunny might have offered her help out of guilt, but things had been progressing between them. She'd even come to like him, in a way. Slowly been opening up, been comfortable enough around him to share the secret of her magic. To do some light apothecary work. The way she'd agreed to help with the delegation plant experiments despite their provenance—surely, that had meant she'd felt... safe?

Certainly, she'd been interested in him enough to look past her guilt. To start to see him as more than her childhood friend. He should've been content with that. Patient. But no, he'd pushed, and now he'd gone too far. All those kindly feelings Eunny held for him? Good chance they were all firmly past tense. In the beginning, she might not have believed herself worthy of his forgiveness, but Ollas and his foolish actions had made sure of it at their end. Rushed her to try her magic, gotten himself injured in the process. Buckled to impatience instead of creating a situation more likely to have success. At so many points leading up to that moment in the greenhouse, he should've chosen different. If only he could try again.

A scoff pushed past his lips. He eschewed the warmth and happiness of the Heartwood, taking the outer stair up to his apartment, his gaze directed at his feet so there was no risk of eye contact and forced pleasantries. Once inside, he shut himself into his room, slumping at his desk. He held his head in his hands.

Try again? He'd do it all the same. Nothing would change. It couldn't. *He* couldn't. He'd been in some kind of love with Eunny since the day they'd met. Objectivity? He didn't know the word. Not when it came to her. Ollas would choose her every time, even when he wasn't wanted. Even when it hurt.

Love you?

The look of pure horror on her face when she'd grasped how serious Ollas was, how he felt about her, it would haunt him for the rest of his days. It would hurt less if she'd taken his quietly confessed love and thrown it back in his face. If she'd laughed, scorned him. Anything but her horrified disbelief. The way she'd looked at him as if seeing the truth for the first time, understood *him* for the first time, and been scared by what she saw.

They held two truths, diametrically opposed. Ollas could never believe she'd want someone like him, and Eunny was repelled by his forgiveness. Couldn't bring herself to accept it. Maybe she would forgive herself once she realized how the fault was shared, or maybe the truth would make her hate him. He'd loved her forever. Couldn't stop, wouldn't even know how to begin. But hurting her? That, he could do something about.

Heaving a sigh, Ollas pulled the short stack of papers he'd brought from his office and set them in the middle of his desk. Graelynd University was looking to fill an adjunct position for its Initiate level botany class. Adjunct pay was shit, but he wasn't exactly high level at Sylveren, either. The prospect of going down to Graelynd didn't appeal, though. It wasn't far enough away, and he didn't relish the thought of going anywhere that might take an interest in his old nickname, even if it was well past being newsworthy.

He flipped to the next letter. His Magister One research was always an option. He could find temporary work in the mountains again as he had during his Adept Two years. The University always had a list of items in need of procurement or transport, and that paid well, too. If he approached the Sentinels, they'd likely take pity on him and find a way to use him, but...no. No, the connection between his old ranger work and the botched rescue was still too close in his head. It would be hard enough to tear himself away without being bombarded with memories of Eunny.

But Ollas couldn't stay here. No matter the outcome. The greenhouse disaster had made him fully realize his bias. Even after all this time, he still wanted to save Eunny. To help her be whole again. Only, she didn't want or need him or his "help." All he did was rip open old wounds, pour salt onto their memories. The kindest thing he could do was let her go instead. Remove himself from the equation.

A knock sounded on his door. Ollas ignored it.

"Olly."

He ignored that, too.

"Ol-*ly*," Gransen's voice lingered in the air.

The mountains sounded good. Gransen had been known to visit Central from time to time, but altitude made him sick. Ollas would find peace there.

"Ollas, I'm coming in. There's nothing I haven't seen before, but for the sake of your delicate sensibilities"—the door opened and Gransen came in, one hand over his eyes—"cover up."

Gransen peeked between his fingers and saw Ollas frowning at him.

"What are you doing here?" Ollas asked.

"I live here, remember?" Gransen walked over and plucked the stack of papers from the desk. "What's this?"

"Granse! Give me that."

The younger man fended him off with his pointy elbow, seating himself upon Ollas's desk. "Did you forget to tell me that you're moving?"

"I'm not in the mood, Gransen."

Something in his voice caused his friend to sit up. Gransen set the papers aside, expression going solemn as he looked Ollas over. "What happened?"

"It's... Eunny and me. We, um, we— I did something." Ollas's sigh turned into a groan. "I hurt her."

Gransen waited.

"She— She trusted me with something, and I took it as something else." Ollas hewed to his side of things, refusing to betray Eunny even more. Those details didn't matter; the core of the problem had always been Ollas. His enthusiasm, his ignoring things like patience or boundaries.

Gransen listened, unspeaking save for the dramatic movements of his brow. When Ollas finished, Gransen sat perfectly still for a moment, chin in hand, eyes squeezed shut.

"Okay, so this does sound kind of bad," he said. He flapped a hand at Ollas when he made a mournful sound. "But it isn't 'pack your bags and move' kind of bad. What's wrong with you? Since when is Ollas Nevin, the Homegrown Hero, a chickenshit?"

"Don't," Ollas growled. "Don't call me that."

"No, we're doing this." Gransen stood up, pointing accusingly at Ollas's chest. "I know that people were annoying about the nickname, but Ollas, you didn't do anything wrong. You didn't then and you haven't now. Whatever happened with Eunny—"

"You weren't there. For any of it. You didn't see—"

"I don't need to see! Because I know you. Whatever happened, you feel worse than you should. Or, you're painting it as worse than it ever could be, because that's who you are, you asshole."

Ollas shook his head. "She probably hates me now."

"She doesn't, and she doesn't mean what she said earlier, either—that stuff you overheard." Gransen sighed. "Just give her a moment. Eun runs a bit hot, you know? But she doesn't actually leave things unsaid. Not important shit."

"Maybe I don't really know her at all. Maybe you don't, either."

Gransen punched him in the shoulder. The still somewhat tender one.

"Ow."

"Earthen take you," Gransen said, exasperated. "Go say you're sorry, and if she's actually going to dump you, make her say it. Or let her, since you're feeling so repentant. But give her a chance to *speak* instead of react." He snatched Ollas's job opportunities from the desk and skipped out of reach.

"Granse!"

"Pity party's over. We'll re-evaluate these if there's a need. A real one. Not while you're still wallowing."

"I don't even— She's not at Belle."

"Ollas." Gransen simply sighed, the sound violent enough to shake his frame. On that enlightening note, he turned around and left.

Ollas stared after his friend. "What the...?"

Eunny was done with him, at least for the moment. Didn't want to see him. Didn't want anything to do with the magic she hated so much.

Gransen had charged him with getting answers. With talking to Eunny, giving her a moment to process that which Ollas had already had the comfort of knowing. She deserved that time, and so did he. Time, and one last try with all honesty bared.

He had to find her.

Where would she go, still reeling from a confrontation with her magic?

Chapter Twenty-Four

BRACING HERSELF FOR THE CREAK, Eunny pushed open the repair café's back door. Even when she'd first opened, it had been heavily scarred, scavenged from another shop down the street. The café's roof collapse had added a few more gouges to the wood, but someone—probably Gransen—had sanded and sealed the damage. Now they added character instead of being a hazard.

The door swung open on quiet hinges. No grumpy squeal of metal or rough scrape of wood improperly set in the frame dragging against the floor. Nothing to remind Eunny that Song's Scrap needed to partake in its own services.

Wariness bumping shoulders with curiosity, Eunny walked inside. Song's Scrap looked...not bad. Even better inside than her brief glimpse through the window. It was a far cry from being fit for the public, but the mess she remembered had been cleared away. A faint scent of mildew remained around the bookshelves, but stronger was the feeling of various cleaning magicks at work. Humidity control charms dangled from the ceiling. The debris had been cleared away and the elements kept out by prodigious use of waxed cloth—Eunny's hasty patch job replaced by one much better. She stopped to touch a length of fabric that was lashed down by the window. Sailcloth from the harbor, and not the cheap stuff. None of the enchantments worked into the fabric were body magic in nature, but the strength of the application tickled her senses all the same.

Eunny turned in a slow circle, struggling to take in the enormity of the changes. The organization, relatively speaking. Things were still broken, both permanent fixtures and backlogged repair jobs, but they weren't in piles scattered all around. No leaky roof or assortment of water-catching vessels scattered around just asking to be tripped over. Some of the old supplies had been lost in the destruction, thus making for less junk to manage in the first place, but Eunny suspected the new, full shelves along the walls were the true reason for order. Those, and the quality of repairs to the café's structure. Not her shitty patch jobs of cut corners and stubbornness.

On the main counter, she found an updated ledger. Orderly script filled the pages: schedules for continued repairs, a list of work orders complete with rough estimates of timeframes and costs, inventory management and multiple contacts noted down for some of the harder-to-obtain items. A separate booklet contained a small calendar with potential dates for a series of "communal cleanup quests" and "a cuppa and a clean."

Gransen had been busy. Not alone, for Eunny spied her aunt's hand in the café's renovations, too, but the self-appointed manager had been up to the task. He'd proven to be a far better custodian of Song's Scrap than Eunny.

But then, why wouldn't he? It was easy to love something when your heart was in it.

Eunny sank onto a stool behind the counter, let her eyes drift around the space. Her repair café. The venture she supposedly cared for enough to put her name on it. Her fresh start, the new life she'd been determined to claim when she'd lost her will for the old one. When she'd escaped the hell of living in Graelynd, in Central, in the same house as her mother. The incessant questions and tests and scornful remarks, all aimed at getting Eunny's magic back. Recovering. Finding it again, as if it was something that had merely fallen from her pocket.

Song's Scrap was proof that she could give up the life she'd known and start over. That she wasn't afraid to do it.

In her head, it had made sense. Open a repair café. She couldn't fix people anymore, so she'd fix things instead, and show that she could do it all without magic. She could do it and be successful and have a life devoid of her magic and her mother. Show that she could be happy. Couldn't she?

Eunny blinked. Tears fell from her eyes. She caught them, her movements automatic, wooden, surprise dulling her brain. When had she started crying? Why was she—

A pointless question. One to which she'd always known the answer—known but carried in silence for so long. Since Song's Scrap had first opened its doors.

She wiped her eyes with the back of her hand, gaze dragging across her surroundings. The café she'd convinced everyone that she loved. Except it was everyone else who loved it. Everyone else who saw Song's Scrap as a Sylvan institution, a beloved fixture in a community notorious for its reticence to welcome outsiders.

There'd been a time when Eunny had been proud of the work her repair café did. She'd been proud of its place here. But she'd never loved it. Perhaps even worse, she didn't hate it either, didn't feel anything so strongly toward it except for *stuck*. Guilty that she'd built this thing so many were invested in, yet she couldn't find that same enthusiasm within herself.

Or was that a lie, too, one she told herself? The guilt was real enough, but the not feeling anything, that wasn't true. Not when it came to Ollas. Apathy wouldn't have made her freeze up in the face of his honesty. If she didn't care, she wouldn't have been so terrified by the prospect of his love. The depth of it. So no, not apathy, but fear and guilt all the same.

She had *run* rather than consider his forgiveness, rather than see if she was finally ready to apply a little to herself. She had broken him; Ollas should've hated her, not been in love. No one had ever put her first like that. She knew her friends and aunt loved her. She had people who cared, people who would drop everything and be there if she needed them. Some would do it if she simply wanted it enough to ask. They were her family. But they also had lives of their own. Wants and dreams that they pursued on their own, and she didn't begrudge them that. Eunny had those things, too, in theory.

Ollas was willing to go further than that. She'd never had someone make her the center of their world. Not even her parents—especially not them—the people who should have come closest to having that kind of a relationship with her. But her father was irrelevant, unknown to all but Bioon, and she'd never seen fit to fill that particular gap in Eunny's knowledge. And of her mother, well... To her mother, Eunny mattered a great deal, but only within the context of what she could do for Bioon's own interests.

Ollas chose her. Loved her. Wanted, *hoped*, she could do the same.

A simple ask, yet with such a cost. *I need you to remember.* The one thing she'd sworn to never do. Relive that day. Remember, as if experiencing it again could change the outcome. It wouldn't. She had quested out with her magic before that day, paired with another's dozens of times without issue. Ollas was still only a victim of her disaster, not the cause.

She'd already done the unthinkable: used her magic. He'd enabled that, had been an encouraging force long before he'd learned the truth of her "lost" power. Because the root of her hatred and sense of betrayal was fear. Ollas softened that fear, made her feel safe, but that safety was a lie. She wasn't safe. Just that minor slip had hurt him. She couldn't be with him, not when she'd be a danger.

Eunny sniffed, tilting her head back to stare at the ceiling. "Sorry, Nev. I can't."

She had started over once. She could do it again. Even if the thought of it hurt a lot more this time.

"There you are." Zhenya stood in the doorway, her entrance inconveniently silent thanks to the now creak-free back door. She looked over her shoulder, calling to someone out of sight, "She's in here."

"Who are you—"

Dae and her younger sister, Calya, filed in after Zhenya.

"What are you doing here?" Eunny asked.

"We could ask you the same question." Dae looked around, finding a wall lamp and turning it up. "Why are you sitting in the dark?"

"I-I'm— I came here because I was..." Eunny stammered, fumbling for the right words. "Sad."

"Why?" Dae and Zhenya chorused, as Calya said, "Very dramatic."

Eunny hesitated. "Because."

Her friends seated themselves around her, concern on their faces. Concern, because... they cared. About her.

Eunny didn't deserve her friends. But she was grateful for them, and they deserved better of her.

"I've been lying to you," she whispered. "About my magic, I —" She raised her hand, palm facing up. Her fingers closed to form a loose fist, then slowly the fist opened, revealing a small handful of light.

No one spoke. Dae and Zhenya exchanged quick looks, as if affirming privately conferred beliefs.

Calya was the one to break the silence, breath coming out as a huff. "So, I'm back to being the only non-magical one?"

Zhenya covered a smile behind her hand as Dae admonished her sister. "Caly!"

Eunny's head swiveled back and forth as she scrutinized each of her friends in turn. "You're—you're not mad? You... *knew?*"

"Suspected," Dae said. "Zhen was the one to figure it out."

Zhenya's cheeks went pink, and her shoulders hunched up around her ears. "I, um, looked at the experiments you and Ollas were running in Trunk. I only looked! I didn't interfere with it at all. But I noticed some traces of light magic in the soil, and it didn't match anything we'd been doing for the elective."

"So you asked Dae? Why didn't you say anything to me?"

Zhenya's shoulders, already hiked up, gave a minute twitch. "You've never wanted to talk about your magic in the first place."

"We figured you had your reasons, for all of it," Dae added. "And, if you ever wanted to tell us, you would."

Eunny gave Calya an expectant look. "How'd you know?"

"I didn't at first, but when I ran into Dae while I was visiting, she had the sample you sent up and was weird about it." Calya's lips formed a thin, smug smile. "I didn't leave until I got answers."

"I could sense your magic in it, too," Dae said. "What I could remember of your magic, anyway. The *cutting,* Eun, it's special. There's definitely healing magic in it."

Eunny gave her a blank look. "Yeah, I got your note. A good preventative—"

"It's more than that. We moved it into soil from a containment zone, and look!" Dae pulled out a sealed vial from her pocket and handed it to Eunny. "Its properties altered when exposed to the higher concentrations of poison. Our sample died, but we were able to work with most of it. The rest is with Ezzyn for testing, but he'll be down here soon."

Eunny squinted at the vial. Inside were dried leaves from a delegation plant, but its veining had a distinct shimmer. "What do you mean? How—"

"Natural augmentative properties. You said the seeds were from the trade delegation? We think they might be Eyllic, or were designed by Eyllic earth mages to react—"

"Much as I love the arcane plant babble, of which I understand nothing," Calya said in a dry tone, "could Eunny remind us again why she was sitting here in the dark?"

"It— It's because of my magic." Eunny tried, failed, to smile. "And Ollas. And my mother." She sighed. "There's a lot of shit going on."

The story spilled out of her, some parts more rushed than others. She didn't linger over the violent rescue or how her magic had damaged Ollas's ability to accept healing. She explained what she could of Zhenya's theory about an imprinting spell on the seeds that still lived on in the plants— that Eunny's last few drops of magic had gone into the seeds, binding them to her and Ollas when her magic lashed out. They already knew how she'd sworn off magic and her apothecary ways. The years of being a magic desert had been easy. If not for the plants' bloom cycle triggering when she came to help Ollas with his teaching duties, she could've lived without magic forever. Only, the plants required more magic to flower, their narrow window to complete the cycle rapidly coming to an end. She confessed her secret uses of magic under Ollas's eye, how she'd thought she'd fooled him, too. The disastrous attempt to push one of the remaining plants to flower, and Eunny's resulting panic. Their fight, if it could be called such a thing.

"An argument, at best," Calya said, nose wrinkling. "Is it really a fight if you both aren't speaking to wound?"

"I was pretty nasty to him," Eunny said, shame-faced.

"Then you were being a jerk—"

"Caly!"

"—but that's not really a fight."

Dae clapped a hand over her sister's mouth. "Keep going," she urged Eunny.

Eunny told them of the theft and catching Bioon in the loft. Her "offer." Its cost if Eunny refused to cooperate.

"People call me a cold-hearted bitch." Calya clucked her tongue. "I'd admire her if she wasn't the enemy."

Dae gave her sister an exasperated look before refocusing on Eunny. "What do you want to do? Whatever it is, we're with you."

The others nodded.

Eunny stared at them. Her lips parted, but emotion clogged her throat. Maybe that was for the best, because it forced her to pause. Look down. Really think about what came next and what she wanted.

And what she didn't.

"I miss my old life. I don't want to be afraid of my magic anymore," she said quietly. "But I'm afraid I'll hurt someone again. How can I use it if my control is so..."

"I can't say for certain, but it might've been the imprinting spell." Zhenya tapped her chin. "Sometimes that kind of spell is used to enforce security measures. It makes sure the goods can't be transferred beyond preset bounds. In this case, you and Ollas."

"Lovely," Eunny said, tone sour. "That sounds like the Coalition."

"Aggressive magic paired with you already spread thin healing everyone from the rescue. That can tip over the strongest mage," Zhenya murmured. "We're most likely to have accidents when fatigued, mentally or physically, and you were both."

"If we're with you, we might be able to help if you feel your-self slipping," Dae said. "You know us, and we don't have the same fear memory that you had with Ollas."

"You're elementalists, though."

"All magic is rooted in light," Zhenya said. "If you have a surge, we'd probably feel it. And it's more about preventing one from happening in the first place."

"We'll be with you the whole way, if that's what you want," Dae said, nudging Eunny's shoulder.

It sounded too easy, based on faith Eunny wasn't sure she shared. Their trust in her was triggering the deep-seated urge to distance herself from such caring.

She forced herself to take a deep breath, hold it, and release at an equally slow pace. She'd said she was tired of being scared. Tired of running. That she wanted the life she'd aban-doned. The life that had lost its spark. Yet, now, that passion had been rekindled, in so many ways. Ollas. She was tired of feeling guilty, of being scared, and using those feelings as reason to deny herself a different future. But those thoughts and words were empty if Eunny wasn't prepared to do some work.

"What do you want to do about the last plant in the mean-time?" Dae asked. "Hide it?"

"If the Coalition already knows about it, then that won't work for long," Calya said. "They have a lot of sway with the Council of Standards."

A faint tugging sensation flared in the back of Eunny's mind. It was a soft, slow gathering of tension, the tiny strands of life in the cutting beginning to pull taut.

Eunny stared at the vial of dried leaves Dae had given her.

They hummed at her. No, they weren't humming. They were *vibrating*, the minute movements creating a whisper against the glass, resonating with a pull coming from further away.

Eunny couldn't say why, but there was a sense of finality to the last cutting stowed somewhere in Trunk and the way it felt in her mind. To her magic.

Her fingers closed protectively around the vial.

Hang on a little longer, baby duck, she thought. *Don't go dying on me now.*

Eunny took another deep breath, rolling her shoulders back as she exhaled. "All right. How do we stop my mother?"

Chapter Twenty-Five

THEY RELOCATED to the back room at the Mighty Leaf. Though Song's Scrap was practically a brand-new place compared to the last time Eunny had seen it up close, it was still far from being comfortable for lengthy visits. Plus, the Mighty Leaf had tea and snacks.

Yerina let the younger women in, promising to drop off a fresh pot and whatever extra pastries she could snag from the displays. Eunny didn't follow the others over the threshold, hesitating as shame burned beneath her skin.

She faced her aunt, raising tentative eyes as she mumbled, "About earlier... What I said. I'm sorry. I—"

Yerina pulled her into a gentle hug. Not her usual, full-bodied, joyful type, but a softer embrace. Tender with emotion, the kind that told Eunny she was still loved despite her aunt's hurt.

"I know." Yerina clasped Eunny's shoulders, holding her at arm's length as she fixed her with a serious look. "But none of that now. We always have later, and you all look...determined."

A dozen replies popped into Eunny's head. Words of fighting, of thwarting Bioon, of prevailing for once, because weren't they due a victory against her scheming? But Bioon was family to them, much as Eunny would rather forget and Yerina would not. Their divergence of opinions on the matter wasn't new, but Eunny's outburst had gone beyond any of their previous disagreements. It was still too fresh, too raw. Deserved more attention and feeling than she could properly give right now. But her aunt knew that, and conveyed her reassurance with a squeeze of her hands.

"We are," Eunny finally said.

"I wouldn't expect any less." Yerina made a shooing motion. "Go on. I'm going to make a pot of the new black spice blend."

"Thanks, Auntie."

Yerina bustled off, and Eunny joined her friends in the back room.

Zhenya had out her notebook crammed full of random inserts and pages covered in her handwriting in multiple colors of ink. She conferred with Dae over a two-page spread while Calya made her own bullet-point list on the back of an old order form.

"What is this?" Eunny joined Zhenya and Dae, twisting around to try and make sense of the drawing from her place across the table.

"It's a flower from my Adept One studies. It didn't work for our intended purposes, but it reminded me of the delegation plants. It had a similar imprinting process spelled into it." Zhenya scanned her notes. "That one did transfer even after propagation. Not very useful for large-scale production if you have a resource locked down to one person."

"Did you figure out how to break the effect?"

"Not during Adept One, and my research ended up changing focus," Zhenya said. "But some Magister levels kept up the work. Professor Rai might be able to put me in contact with them."

"Worth a shot," Eunny said, grim-faced. "Not fast enough for my current problem, though."

"You're probably not alone in this, whether you like it or not," Dae said slowly. "There are records of the sample I took back to Rhell, and the Restorers are interested in growing more."

"If it can be brought to seed," Zhenya said. Dae gave a conceding nod. "Which still needs you, Eunny."

"Which would rope me in with the Rhellian government. Possibly the Order of Sylveren, or at very least the university, since I used school materials for my experiments," Eunny said. "I've had worse bedfellows."

"Better to not be the sole target when dealing with the Coalition," Calya piped up. "It's nice when you can spread the blame."

Eunny fingered the vial in her pocket, the dried leaves sliding along the glass. "Yeah, the Coalition is shit when it comes to sharing."

"Good luck to them," Dae muttered. "If the plant can help save Rhell, then Ez will go to war to keep it." She looked to Zhenya. "All right, so we're back to you getting your last cutting to complete its life cycle. Are there better storage options if we need to smuggle the seeds out in a hurry?"

"I can look into something with more protection enchants," Zhenya replied. "I'll head back to the Grove and see what I can put together."

Eunny glanced at the room's small wall clock and winced. "Bioon will be back in the morning. Probably early, knowing her."

"I'll work fast," Zhenya promised.

The remaining trio settled in for a long night, the Helm sisters rebuffing Eunny's concern.

"Hardly my first all-nighter," Calya said. "And I love beating the Coalition at their own game. It happens so rarely."

"We might not," Eunny warned. "Will HNE's trustee be okay with this? It's not really applicable to the shipping business."

"As far as Mr. Wembly is concerned, I'm up here tidying accounts after the mess Brint made." Calya's shoulders lifted with an indifferent shrug. "My work for Helm Naval's been done. How I spend my recreational time is my business, and Mr. Wembly can report that to Andrin."

"Caly," Dae said, her tone long-suffering. "You really shouldn't call Papa that."

Calya rolled her eyes. She started to respond, but it was interrupted by the door opening to admit a tall man with long, pale blond hair, his travel leathers splashed with mud.

"Ez!" Dae jumped up to greet her partner.

Ezzyn bent to kiss her, his hands filled with a heavily laden tea tray. He murmured his thanks when Eunny relieved him of it, then dropped into Zhenya's vacated seat with a grateful sigh.

"I left about a day behind you, give or take a few hours," he said in answer to Dae's unspoken question. "Took a windrunner from the Lower Sohn here."

"What happened with your testing?" Dae asked.

"That's why I rushed here." Ezzyn looked around at all of them. "When we exposed the plant to containment zone soil, it's like it restructured itself internally. The grovetenders haven't seen anything like it."

"Does it neutralize the poison?" Eunny asked, hope welling in her chest.

He shook his head. "It grew well, but it doesn't have a restorative effect on its own." He leaned forward. "The plant itself, though, it definitely works for healing augmentation that *can* cleanse the sickness in people if they're treated early. The cutting you sent, it had traces of the Valley in it, the way magic feels here. It's hard to explain, and we need to run more tests, but it seems like we can attune—"

"What does all of that mean?" Calya interrupted. "For those of us who don't speak arcane."

Dae and Ezzyn talked over one another as they tried to give examples Calya would understand.

Eunny paid attention with only half an ear, turning this latest information over in her mind. The scattered morsels of ideas she'd been acquiring for the last couple months began to coalesce.

Seeds that grew well, even *thrived* in the blighted soil of Rhell. Plants that amplified healing magic, that could be personalized, like the healing draught Dae had received at the Healing Hut. Those plants could—maybe—be vessels for the kind of magic that withstood the poison. A merging of the protection inherent in the Valley and the plants' response, altering their form when grown in the blight.

Ezzyn turned to Eunny, pulling a folded slip of paper from his pocket and handing it to her. "I almost forgot—your aunt said this was left for you."

She quickly scanned the page, eyebrows rising as she took in the hastily written words. "It's from Ollas. He heard back from Nocren, the Sentinel who's been liaising with the Coalition. Says that they've been forwarding all the reports from Ollas and Rai and the samples from the elective to some rural site out in Desmond's Landing."

"Desmond's Landing," Dae murmured, confusion clouding her face as she thought. "Why does that sound... Oh! Caly, isn't that where Brint's shady side project was held? The one that got him in trouble with the Coalition and the board for Avenor Guard?"

"Brint?" Eunny said, naming Dae's ex-fiancé, Calya's ex-business partner, and overall human waste of space.

Calya frowned. "Possibly. The protection route went to the lower river rather than up to the Landing. But, there's not much out there. Isn't it protected forestland?"

"He was trying to cover up a problem with an environmental project," Dae said slowly, squinting as she tried to dredge up memories. "That was why he came to Sylveren last year, to try to scam some grovetenders into helping him."

"What does that have to do with the Coalition, though?" Eunny asked. "Why would they send class reports out to the middle of nowhere?"

Her words were met with shrugs.

"Maybe they're hoping to scoop the school and bring a working version of the plant to market first?" Dae suggested.

"They're sponsoring the elective. I'm pretty sure the school's justiciars would—"

"Worry about that after you have your own plant in hand," Calya said. "Now, then. Presuming all this success is repeatable, what's next?"

"If we can push a new generation of seeds, I'll need to get them to Rhell right away if the Coalition is on the hunt," Eunny said. "We're talking greater good, here—think I should see if the university will help? They might call on the Sentinels to facilitate some safe passage."

"There are HNE windrunners with the latest hull enhancements in port at Renstown," Calya said. "I can arrange for one to be reassigned."

"You will want to talk to the school eventually, or maybe even the Order," Dae said, gaze going unfocused as she stared off in thought. "We're looking at multiple cross-border dealings. Growing the plants in Rhell, infusing the leaves with healing magic in the Valley, and then transporting them back to Rhell... Caly?"

"Our riverboats can handle the Lower Sohn waterways," Calya said. "That segment of the fleet is down, though, and lumber prices are terrible right now. If you're talking premium speed enchantments, the wood required for that is niche."

"A deal can be struck with the Rhellian government," Ezzyn said. "There's also the Restorers. This fits their mission statement perfectly."

Calya was making notes on a fresh piece of paper as they talked. She glanced at Eunny. "You're going to be busy, assuming this works."

Eunny stared at the paper and Calya's underlined groupings. Helm Naval Engineering. The Rhellian government. Potential funding from the Restorers of the Alliance. Partner work with the appropriate departments at Sylveren. Though she'd been thinking out loud for hours, Eunny hadn't really processed the implications and what they would mean for her. She hadn't thought beyond having to willfully use her magic. Which was significant, given her aversion, but it wasn't the only substantial change. She'd have to shepherd the new seeds to Rhell. See them into the ground, maybe even help them grow. What if the plants' transition to new caretakers didn't go well and she had to stay in Rhell for a while? No more swinging by to help Auntie Yerina at the tearoom, at least not for a bit. She'd have to close Song's Scrap. No point in getting the repair café fixed up only to be put on hiatus for an undetermined amount of time.

And Ollas, what of him? He had his teaching and a life here in Sylvan. Eunny knew herself well enough that asking for long-distance was asking for failure.

She took the vial of dried leaves from her pocket, reaching with a whisper of magic, just enough to feel the inherent thread of light humming in response to her nudge. To think that this had all started with a selfish wish to ease only her guilty mind. Now she was considering getting tied up with multiple nations and big-time organizations, all to best her mother. Well, and because it was the right thing to do. Both—it was both, and if Eunny derived more satisfaction from one than the other, who cared so long as good was served in the end.

"Yeah," she said, voice faint. "Things are going to have to change around here."

"I've got messages to send." Calya stood. "The Coalition will have to pass through Renstown. I'll see if I can stall them."

"Carefully, Caly. If Wembly—"

"Stop mothering me, Anadae." Calya stuck her tongue out at her sister. "I was born for this."

"Brat." Dae hugged her, ignoring her feeble struggle.

Eunny met Calya's eye. "I'll owe you one."

"Don't I know it. One of these days, I'll come to collect."

Once the door had closed again, Eunny snagged a pastry from the neglected tea tray. She scooted her chair next to Dae's, and they began compiling a list of next steps.

A gentle shake of her shoulder roused Eunny from sleep. She groaned, her neck and back protesting as she tried to straighten. There was a weight about her shoulders. A blanket. One she didn't recognize.

Blinking heavy eyes, she peered around the darkened room. "What time is it?"

"Almost dawn."

Eunny spun around. Tried to, anyway. She was too old for this shit, falling asleep anywhere that wasn't a bed—she tweaked her back in the process and only made a partial turn before she abandoned the attempt and filled the air with a chorus of "fuck" through gritted teeth.

"Here." A mug of fresh, steaming tea was placed in front of her.

She took a greedy sip, moaning in appreciation as a hint of lemon zipped across her tongue. She dipped her finger inside the mug, letting it kiss the surface as she called up a dot of light. Just a little something to ease some of the tightness from her muscles. The next sip helped, and by the third swallow, she felt vaguely human again. The small bit of magic wasn't much, but it had come back to her, still second nature even if its potency was lacking.

Though the sleepy haze was clearing, her mind was far from empty. The restless feeling was back, the call of the last plant and its need for her magic to complete its life cycle. The thought made a hum of magic dance across her fingertips.

More awake now, she remembered that she wasn't alone.

"Nev?" she said, goggling at him. A soft smile tugged at the corners of his mouth, but tension remained. Quiet hope and apprehension in equal measure cast a shadow on his face.

The old guilt rose up again in Eunny's gut, doubt restraining her newfound resolve as some of his hesitation rubbed off on her. "Where— When..."

She'd fallen asleep in the back room. Dae was stirring from where she'd slept, similarly hunched over in her seat at the table. Ezzyn was gone.

"A little while ago. Ezzyn filled me in," Ollas said, handing Dae a mug of tea. "We thought it best to give you another hour."

"Before?" Eunny rubbed her eyes, mind clicking along a beat behind. "Why are we awake at this godsforsaken—"

Almost dawn. The windrunner schedule from Renstown

across the lake would have the early ones in around daybreak. Bioon was coming.

Her eyes met with Ollas. "Oh, shit. I've— *We've* got to go." She looked at Dae. "The cutting."

Dae blinked a few times, then sat bolt upright. "I'll find Zhenya." She stumbled from the room.

Eunny moved to follow, then stopped. Ollas was right next to her, so close she could feel the tension as he held himself back.

"Nev," she whispered. "I— I'm so shit at this. I'm sorry." Godsdamned mother*fuck*. Eunny knew that she had flaws, that serious relationships might as well be foreign concepts to her. She knew they'd have plenty of "couple" things to work out. Most of all, though, Eunny knew she was done being a chicken-shit about how much she wanted Ollas.

Eunny's shoulders jerked with a weak laugh as she gave him a small, nervous smile. "I'm sorry, and I know there should be more and we should have an actual conversation like grown adults and be, you know, *responsible* or something—"

Ollas gently cupped her face, relief making his voice crack as he murmured, "It's okay."

"It's not!" Eunny insisted. "But the proper make-up will have to wait till later, because I have to go possibly commit some crime and stop my mother."

"Ezzyn mentioned that." Ollas rested his forehead against hers. "I'm here. Whatever you need, I'm here."

"What about your job? This will probably go against your contract with Sylveren—"

"Eunny." Ollas silenced her with a kiss. "I made my choice."

Her lips reached for him again even as she tried to protest. "But—"

"It's who I am." He stepped back, holding on only to the tips of her fingers. He offered a smile, but it was a wistful one.

Sportsmanlike, admitting defeat with grace. "I choose you. I love *you*, Eunny, and I'd choose you over a job every time."

"Ollas."

He shook his head. "Don't. You don't have to say anything, Not now, never, if you don't want to. Just know that's how I feel. Always have."

Gods all break. It was too early for her to be feeling so many things and have so many important decisions to make when she didn't have the time or brain power to process any of them to the fullest.

For some things, she had to go on instinct.

Eunny slid her hand forward so that it firmly held his, lacing her fingers through his own.

"You know, if people are going to call you a hero"—she smoothed the frown lines from his brow—"we might as well make the most of it. I don't need rescuing, but I could use your help. Will you keep me safe, Ollas?"

Eunny saw a new smile light his face—beaming, one might call it—for only a second before his mouth was on hers again. A tremble ran through him, relief and delight and echoes of the hunger she remembered from their first kiss the night she'd moved into her own place. He wanted her, of that there was no doubt. And, for the first time, Eunny let herself bask in the realization without a hint of shame. She let her fingers slide through his curls and hold him close because he was *hers*.

"What do you need?" he murmured against her lips.

"What did you do with the last cutting?"

"It's in Trunk. I wasn't sure what— If you were coming back." He grimaced. "I figured the thieves already thought they got everything and wouldn't come back, but I stashed it in the rear antechamber."

"Then that's where we need to go." She tapped her temple,

as if she could almost grab hold of the pulling sensation. "Can you feel it, too?"

Ollas nodded slowly. "The bloom window. It's fading."

Dae dashed back into the room, a piece of paper clutched in her fingers. "Calya says your mother is coming in early."

With Ollas in tow, Eunny headed for the door. "Dae, can you find Zhen? Forget about helping with the seeds, we'll figure something out." She jerked her thumb to indicate Ollas. "Zhen will know about getting the right dirt to get us to Rhell."

"Soil," Ollas whispered.

"Got it. Ez can help." Dae ran off.

Eunny was nearly out of the tearoom when she saw her aunt replacing stock at the front counter. Leaving Ollas to wait, she approached Yerina.

"Auntie," Eunny said quietly. "I need to ask you something."

Slowly, Yerina turned around, her normally cheery face now solemn.

"I know we don't agree on... on anything to do with my mother," Eunny said. "I never should've said she hates you. I didn't mean it. I just... I don't know why you try so hard for her, either. She'll never—"

"She's my sister. That still means something to me," Yerina said, her voice soft. She reached out to hold Eunny's hand. "But that's my decision. It shouldn't influence how you feel about her, or how you want your relationship with her to be."

"I hate her." Eunny's lip trembled. "I'm sorry, but I do. I'm sorry, Auntie."

Yerina's face softened, grief and love in equal measure in her smile. "Don't be. You get to decide what that relationship is worth."

"You won't be mad at me?" Eunny said. "Or think I—"

"Never, Eunji." Yerina hugged her, so tightly that her back cracked. "Oh, I'm sorry, dear."

"No, I think you got it back how it's supposed to be," she wheezed. "Listen, Auntie, if my mother comes here looking for me..."

"I can't lie to her."

"I know, I just... If you could—"

"But I can ask her to listen," Yerina continued. "I haven't asked anything of her in a long time. That won't be worth much"—her smile turned sad again—"but it could be a little."

"Good enough for me."

Kissing her aunt on the cheek, Eunny raced back to Ollas and pulled him out the door.

Chapter Twenty-Six

At such an ungodly hour, the university's grounds were deserted. Across the courtyard, Eunny picked out movement; a few people could be seen inside the elementalists' Towers through the atrium's massive glass windows. The Heartwood was softly aglow, too, though no sound drifted outward as Eunny and Ollas hurried past. Everything was lit in the bluish cast of pre-dawn, dark but not so dark that they couldn't see the path as they ran to the furthest of the six greenhouses. Eunny had made the journey so many times by now she figured she could do it in her sleep. Nervous energy made her hand shake as she pulled open the greenhouse door. What if they couldn't get the cutting to flower? Or worse, got it to flower but not set seed, and then her mother showed up with enough Coalition muscle to take the plant by force? Tinkering with her magic when she was tired, stressed… Her control was already questionable. If the imprinting spell kicked up, if she panicked again, if—

Ollas gave her hand a gentle squeeze. "It'll be fine. I know you can do this."

Eunny cracked a weak smile. "Or I'm about to fry—"

He took her chin between his fingers, muffling her words with his lips. "Don't even think it." He released her and went to turn the interior lamps to their lowest setting. "I'll get fresh soil."

"I'll grab the plant."

Eunny ducked into the rear antechamber. The cutting was tucked behind several larger plants, safe in its small jar. When she grabbed it, an electric tingle zipped over her fingers as the leaves stretched against their glass walls. The tugging in her head intensified for a moment, causing her eye to twitch.

"Stop it," she whisper-admonished, heading back into the greenhouse's main room. "I'm going, all right?"

She watched Ollas portion out some amendment and give it a proper mix with blighted dirt. Eunny hoped it would be enough, that it would matter at all. Help, in some small way, so feeding the plant didn't rest solely on her. On them. If she'd learned anything from her time at the Grove, it was a greater respect for the amount of energy a plant put into flowering. Accelerating the process would demand more magic than she'd used in a long time. Six years. She hadn't lost her magic in a literal sense, but the practiced ability to maintain steady energy and control, *that* would have lapsed. The raw source was still within her, but she remembered all too well how magic could escape when one's control was low. How magic could *take*. True, she'd been exhausted when the imprinting spell was first activated, her inner well drained practically dry, her mind too sapped to put up much of a fight when those seeds had called. But she'd been more practiced then. Confident. Willing to call herself a mage, a mender, rather than a fake mundane trying to be handy and crafty.

Ollas scooted a clay pot full of soil mix in front of her. "Ready?"

Eunny put her hand on the jar, fingers hesitating over the cork lid.

"No," she admitted. "But I don't really have a choice, do I?"

"You do," Ollas said. "We can leave for Rhell right now, and there's the—"

She shook her head. "It won't make it." She rubbed the glass with a finger. The veins on the cutting's leaves were starting to glow with a faint, flickering light. "Besides. Running and hiding? I think I've done that long enough."

"What can I do?" he asked.

She offered up her hand. "Keep me grounded."

He hesitated, his fingers curled away from her even as his palm hovered above. "Eunny…"

She reached out to graze her fingertips across his cheek. "I remembered. Nev, you didn't make me lose control. Menders tap into others' light all the time in practice."

His head bowed. "The seeds were in my pocket when I reached out. If I hadn't done that, we never would've triggered the imprinting spell. It's my fault."

Eunny cupped his face between her hands. "It's not. Neither of us could've known." When his gaze remained downcast, she gave him a small shake. "I forgive you, Nev, okay? Can you accept that?"

Ollas turned his head so he could press a kiss against the palm of her hand. "If you can accept mine."

"Deal." Eunny took a step back and offered her hand again. "Ready?"

Ollas laced his fingers through hers. "Yes, but I'm not sure what we're supposed to do."

"You're the grovetender, *Professor.* If you notice me going off into the weeds, do something teacherly."

Eunny reached for a thread of her light, mentally taking hold against the increasingly familiar pull as the magic tried to reach for the cutting. She gently rubbed one of the cutting's leaves between her thumb and forefinger, letting her magic go. The glowing line of light coursed from her fingers into the glossy green leaf, filling the stems and branches as it followed the pull down into the soil. The veining in the leaves went from a flickery shine to a blaze of gold.

Eunny tensed as her flow of magic surged. Panic welled up as she fought the plant for control, instinctively resisting the pull.

"It's okay," Ollas murmured. "It needs the energy. Just don't let it boss you around."

She exhaled, her breath coming in long and shaky gasps, but she let more of her power go in a steady stream. She kept her mental touch firm but not restrictive as the cutting drank up their magic. She could feel the plant filling, magic accumulating within it as if the plant was a vessel. It left her with a vague yet satisfying impression, as if the veins of each leaf, once sufficiently filled, dropped to the back of her awareness like boxes ticked on a checklist.

When the last leaf was full, the flow of magic abruptly reversed. A strange current zipped back up to burst along Eunny and Ollas's joined hands. Eunny yelped, more out of surprise than actual pain from the shock, but she dropped Ollas's hand as she jumped back.

"Nev!" she immediately ran her hands over him, across his face, down his chest, questing out with her magic for any sign of injury. "Are you okay?"

He laughed, catching her hands and dropping his head to give her a reassuring kiss. "Yes. I'm fine, love."

"What the fuck was that?" she asked, frowning at her hand and shaking it to remove the phantom tingle from being shocked.

"I think it's the imprinting spell." Ollas peered intently at his hand, calling up a weak spark of his own magic as he probed one of the leaves. "The way the spellwork was laid into the plant... I've never seen anything like it. We don't apply enchantments like that here."

They both looked down at the pot. The plant hadn't grown up so much as out, its leaves so thick they almost looked swollen. It burst with dozens of deep pink buds the size of her thumbnail.

Eunny puffed her cheeks out. "Well, that's disappointing. I was hoping for a bit more drama. Fit the mood."

Ollas snorted, kissing her again before gesturing toward the plant. "Look at the buds."

The tightly furled, immature blooms were lit from within, the intensity wavering with tiny pulses like a heartbeat.

She nudged one with a glowing fingertip. It didn't grow, but it and the other blossoms hummed in response. She could sense traces of her and Ollas's magic in each bud. The nascent bloom's essence had a malleable quality, a sponge-like feeling to her magic, eager to absorb. The pulling sensation she'd been resisting for months, the feeling of restless certainty, emanated from each tiny flower-to-be. When she fed in just a drop of her magic, the bud immediately sucked it up. This time, unlike when she'd tested the handful of seeds six years ago, she felt a soft plucking motion at the edge of her mind, as if the bud was incomplete.

"They're Eyllic," she murmured.

Though she didn't look away from the plants, Eunny felt Ollas turn beside her in question.

"I was brought along for the delegation to check the veracity of some goods supposedly being negotiated for the deal. But really, my mother wanted me to see if these were legitimate healing plants." She glanced at Ollas. "But why would the Coalition want seeds for a plant that can only act as a preventative for the poison? Dae and Ezzyn didn't work out their containment wards until years later. They couldn't have known then that we'd have a way to control the spread at the expense of making the corruption stronger."

"She wanted you to test the seeds… Seeds that had a strong imprinting spell enchanted into them," Ollas said slowly.

"Do you think the imprinting spell was meant to keep the supply restricted?"

"At least at first. Their bloom cycle has some unique parameters," Ollas said with a wry smile. "You did say that the Coalition only cares about profit. Even as a preventative, these plants are valuable."

But engaging in self-serving trade like that with the Eyllics during wartime wasn't allowed. The rest of the Empyrean Territories would've blasted Graelynd for encouraging profiting off a humanitarian crisis like that. Eunny wasn't versed in the terms of the alliance between the nations, but she guessed that monetizing potential cures, not to mention using the trade delegation as a front for those shady dealings, went against the agreements the Territories had with each other. And it wasn't even Graelynd doing it, but the Coalition.

The Coalition who'd orchestrated the delegation. Who'd gone to great lengths to recover the strange plants. Bioon hadn't seemed bothered by Eunny's reveal that the plants were dying. The Coalition had trashed the records regarding the seeds, stolen what they'd thought were the remainders of the plants. Bioon, who'd shown up on behalf of the Coalition to have an interest in the elective. Who had Ollas and Rai supplying progress reports at a ridiculous rate, which were then being sent off to some random corner of rural Graelynd. Her mother, who came with her fucking threats disguised as a deal. So many parts, yet none of them fit together in a way that made sense. It needled at Eunny, but the last piece refused to come clear.

"Have you heard about anyone else taking notice of these plants?" Eunny asked. "Aside from Zhen."

Ollas shook his head. "Rai knew I was dabbling, but they're unrelated to the work we're doing with the elective, so we didn't discuss it much. Or, they *were* unrelated, but Ezzyn mentioned the way they change in heavily poisoned ground, and those could be interesting—"

The sound of footsteps pounding toward the greenhouse caused them both to look up. Bioon, flanked by two men in combat leathers, appeared in the doorway. Dressed all in black, her expression a cold mask—Eunny could see why her mother was known informally as the Scourge of the Coalition. Bioon strode forward, exuding arrogance with every step. "Eunji, give me that plant and—"

There'd be no reasoning with her, not while Bioon viewed the greenhouse as yet another domain she'd conquered.

But in all the frenzied hours Eunny and her friends had spent strategizing, reasoning with Bioon had never been part of the plan.

Eunny glanced at Ollas. He gave her a tiny nod. "Go!"

Chapter Twenty-Seven

Ollas pulled Eunny toward the rear antechamber, the one that had housed their secret seed project all term. She grabbed their potted cutting, now the size of a small shrub and bursting with unopened buds, and scrambled inside.

Ollas slammed the door shut behind her. Then, hitting a rune emblazoned on the wall, he locked them in together.

Ushering Eunny toward the back of the antechamber, Ollas faced the door. Eunny's mother appeared in the half-window. The door handle rattled when she tried it, but it didn't budge.

"Open the door, Mr. Nevin," Bioon said. "Do not make this worse for yourself."

"Says the thief." Eunny came up beside him. She stared at her mother as if seeing her in a new, unflattering light. "What are you doing, Mother? There's no sneaking off into the dark this time. The school will know what you've done, and so will the Sentinels."

"True, but I have a job to do, Eunji." Bioon's arm moved, but the door hid her hand from view. "A duty, and you would see my point of view if your judgment about the Coalition wasn't so clouded."

Ollas stepped away from the door, scanning the wall. The greenhouses weren't exactly armories, and when it came to tools that could serve as weapons, the antechambers were even more lacking than the central room. The long-handled hoes and big shears hanging on the other side of the wall would've come in handy right about now. Even worse, Trunk was just the storage building. No fancy, blade-like protector plants in here.

"You threatened your own sister and her business, but I'm the one with the shit judgment?" Eunny said, incredulous. "You want to steal the thing that could help save Rhell!"

"They're effective against the poison, then? Those plants are Coalition property, and as such, the organization will see to their distribution. An organization that keeps a *nation* prosperous can't be sentimental."

"They're not Coalition property, though," Eunny said slowly, gaze going distant as she thought. "You had me check them at the delegation. They're Eyllic."

Bioon's expression went carefully neutral.

"Why was the Coalition negotiating for plants effective against the poison? If you were there to bargain over something like that, Rhell should've been involved."

"It was a complex situation, and it wasn't necessary for you to be privy to all of the topics being discussed," Bioon said with a dismissive shake of her head.

"How did you even know about them?" Eunny asked. "Now. Here."

"The Coalition has been monitoring the elective's progress closely. Its successes have great implications for the market—"

"I've never mentioned them," Ollas said, earning a withering look from the older woman. "Neither has Rai. These aren't part of the elective at all."

"And you didn't start asking questions until later," Eunny said, more to herself than either of them. She met Ollas's eyes.

"After *you* started looking into the greenhouse records. That must've tipped them off, because she ambushed me at the Mighty Leaf, was asking if I remembered anything about the delegation. Wanted to know if the elective had started a new trial, and asked me to report on you. Like I'd ever do that for you." She directed the latter statement at her mother with a derisive scoff.

Bioon's eyes closed briefly, nostrils flaring with an annoyed sigh. Just as quickly, her eyes snapped back open, fixing on her daughter. "I warned you not to meddle in the Coalition's affairs." She glanced to her left, chin dipping in a small nod at one of the guards standing next to her before her gaze flicked back to Eunny. "I *did* tell you that."

"Watch out," Ollas said, reaching for Eunny as the butt of a garden hoe's wooden shaft slammed into the window.

"Shit." Eunny staggered back a step. A round indent had formed in the glass, small cracks fanning out around it.

Bioon held up a hand to stop the guard from attacking again. She met Eunny's eyes, her expression impassive. Like this was business as usual, regardless of the conditions. Then again, Ollas was beginning to think she really did feel that way.

"Last chance," she said. "This door won't hold. Hand over the plant and I'll ensure Rhell gets first call on the product, at cost."

Eunny held up the pot and gave it a taunting shake. "Liar. This thing would be up in flames before we left the building."

Bioon turned to Ollas. "And you, Mr. Nevin? The Coalition will press charges over your handling of its property. You won't have a teaching position here anymore if you continue to stand against us."

"I like where I'm standing," Ollas said. "Ma'am."

"Fucking shameless," Eunny muttered.

Bioon heaved a disgusted sigh. She stepped back again, motioning for her guard to continue breaking down the door.

"This isn't Graelynd," Eunny said. "The Coalition has no authority here. You won't get away with this, Mother." From the corner of her mouth, she muttered, "Any ideas, Nev?"

Another blow to the glass sent cracks spreading nearly the full width of the window. The grovetender-made glass was strong, laced with enchantments, but it hadn't been crafted with the intention of keeping intruders out. Ollas batted one of the spindly vines out of his way as he searched for something, *anything* that could help. Sylveren was a civilian school, not a military—

His eyes followed the path of the sparse vines tracing the upper edges of the antechamber. They grew along the ceiling, only trailing down to the floor in a few places, like the corners of the small room. A single strand had traveled down to trace the edge of the doorframe. The vine was still spindly, still had smallish leaves—and not very many of them at that—but it wasn't quite so dry and flaky thanks to Ollas's recent efforts to nourish it. He never had managed to find the mother stem's pot, but at this point, the plant seemed to have spread throughout Trunk and drawn bare sustenance from every available source. True, it was nowhere near as impressive as what Rai kept in his office; certainly not as big or resilient as the ones living in Sprout. Not much worth protecting in the storage greenhouse, after all. But it was still alive, still one of the school's protective measures.

If only Ollas had a handful of magic to offer the dormant plant.

Eunny and her mother were yelling at each other through the glass. Their sharp words were nearly drowned out by the guard battering away at the window, chunks of glass ripping free and crashing to the floor. Ollas ignored them all, going to the wall and reaching out to touch the vine where it came down next to the door. He willed a few sparks of light to his fingers, holding his breath as they settled atop the vine. His magic rested there, in particles so small they could've been mistaken for motes of dust if not for their arcane gleam. The dots didn't wink out, but they weren't absorbed into the vine's woody exterior, either.

"No authority." Bioon laughed, the sound high-pitched. Cold. "Oh, Eunji, you think this godsforsaken place has power? Control of commerce, *that* is real power. The world revolves around money, whether you like it or not. Your precious Valley cannot exist on morals alone. You speak of authority? The Coalition ensured the end of a war. The Order of Sylveren couldn't achieve that."

"Funny, I don't remember the Coalition sailing a fleet it doesn't have up to fight the Empire."

"Who do you think convinced Graelynd's navy to sail?" Bioon asked in a falsely sweet tone.

"The Upper Council. They voted after the delegation." Eunny faltered, eyes widening. "After the— After we— Oh, that's rich, taking credit for us getting kidnapped. What, did you plan that, too?"

"What?" Ollas blurted. He realized he'd been watching their exchange, Bioon's revelation shocking him to a standstill. His attention was torn between the women and the vines as he reached for more of his magic; it gurgled in him, weak as ever, his drops of light more like soap bubbles and just as apt to pop.

"The Coalition organized the delegation," Eunny said without looking at him. She glared at her mother, though, at this point, it was difficult to see Bioon through the fractured glass.

"You forget that none of us were pleased by the Eyllics' treachery." Bioon sniffed. "The war was hurting trade. Everywhere, not just for Graelynd, but the Councils didn't act until their own people were mistreated. We didn't plan it, but the Coalition certainly helped the Councils make the correct decision."

The specks of Ollas's magic were gone now. He reached inward, trying to visualize his inner well as all the textbooks and instructions he'd scoured always said. But he'd come to realize long ago that his well was always on the dry side. Unfortunately, adrenaline didn't lend him any strength in this regard.

Desperate, he grabbed the vine and shook it. Nothing happened. No surge of power beneath his fingers, no explosion of sparks. Their options hadn't been good when they'd escaped into the antechamber, he'd known that, but he had always been something of an optimist. Full of hope.

Regret twisted in his chest; he'd failed Eunny, failed to keep her safe when she'd asked it of him.

Ollas cast about for any sort of weapon. Plenty of projectiles in the form of potted plants, though they'd be unwieldy. The reed sticks serving as plant stakes were laughable in comparison to whatever garden tools Bioon's henchmen were armed with, but they'd have to do. Ollas pulled one from a large plant near the back wall.

"Eunny," he rasped, preparing to step between her and her mother, "take the plant. You have to—"

The guard succeeded in breaking the glass, the butt of a long shovel crashing through with an explosion of shards. He jerked the wooden pole from side to side, clearing away the jagged pieces that remained in the window frame. The other guard stepped forward and reached inside, searching for the rune carved into the wall and—

Every hair on Ollas's arms stood up. An electric crackle zipped through the air and sped across his skin before vanishing. It left him staggering in its wake. The sensation was incorporeal yet so powerful he felt it in his bones.

Vines dropped from the ceiling, latching on to the door.

One landed on the guard's arm, startling a yell from him. Everywhere the vines made fresh contact, they sent out aerial roots, digging into wood, grasping every surface. The guard cursed, fighting to extract his arm from the roots.

A vine brushed against Eunny's sleeve, immediately catching the fabric. She yelped, trying to jerk her arm back. Ollas grabbed the vine with one hand and Eunny with the other, desperation granting him one more tiny spark of light. The vine let go, the new greenish roots loosening as they wavered in the air, searching for new purchase.

Ollas hauled Eunny back until they were clear of the vines wriggling in the air.

"What did you do?" she whisper-shouted.

"I think it's protecting the greenhouse," he replied, awestruck as more vines fell across the broken window, slowly creating a barrier of thick, tough stems.

"What happened to plants not being sentient enough for malice?"

"*Most.* I said most."

On the other side of the living wall, Bioon could be heard yelling at the guards to find axes. Ollas tried to listen—better to have an idea of their next move—but a strange hum built in his ears. The hairs on his nape prickled as a phantom hand all but pushed him toward the potted plant still clutched in Eunny's hands.

The hum shifted, became more of a ringing sound that grew louder with each pulse of his heart. Not sweet and bell-like but an unpleasant, sheer noise that sent minute vibrations coursing down his body. His inner sphere of light, though weak, popped and fizzed in response, causing erratic blips of magic to flare at his fingertips.

"Eunny, the bloom cycle." Ollas drew her back to the antechamber's far corner. "I don't think we have much time. You're going to need to give it a push." He cleared a space for her pot on the upper rack.

Eunny set it down, a sad smile on her face as she gave one of the pink buds a gentle pat. "I don't know if I have enough magic left."

"I can guide you. I think. If you'll let me," he murmured. "Just enough for the transfer, then I'll drop off and—"

"No." Eunny bit her lip, indecision in her eyes. Slowly, she held her hand out to him. "It imprinted on both of us. I think it *needs* the both of us. Can you feel it?"

Ollas touched one of the leaves, eyes closing as a flicker of his light eagerly shot into the plant. A certain tension seeped into the air, seemed to wrap around the plant and cause its leaves to curl at the edges. A pressure built in Ollas's head.

"The imprinting spell," he said.

"Nev, you'll probably be tied to these again until we figure out how to pass it on or break it or whatever," Eunny murmured. "It could be years, if we're stuck with this bloom cycle thing. It'll definitely complicate things for your teaching."

Bioon's threats of pressing charges and costing Ollas his job lingered at the back of his mind. Even if she was bluffing, Eunny was probably right; he'd be locked in for whatever the seeds entailed. His grand return to Sylveren and teaching again would be disrupted, and he hadn't even been back a full year.

But he wouldn't be in it alone.

"I choose you, remember?" Ollas took her hand. "Every time."

∿

Trust didn't come easily for Eunny. Not with a mother like she had. Some of that was on her. She trusted so few, and even those people, she barely let them in. She let in Dae and Zhenya. Trusted them, loved them. They were her family and would protect her if she let them. She had in some ways. But in other ways, maybe she didn't because it had never felt quite right.

With Ollas, those subconscious barriers fell away. He was safe. Everything about him: the warmth of his hand in hers, the sputtery little drop that was his magic, the sensation in Eunny's mind when her magic curled around his and coaxed it to join; all of it came together in her mind. The prospect of giving him such intimate access, something far more profound than just her body—for once, Eunny didn't feel any trepidation. Didn't feel any guilt for handing over this part of herself. Didn't feel any guilt over being willing to bond, with all of the joys and burdens it entailed.

She was making Ollas responsible, at least in part, for whatever actions her magic wrought, good and bad. And she didn't feel the least bit anxious about it.

Maybe that was love—feeling comfortable enough with someone that you gave them some of your mess. It was the height of intimacy. Or selfishness. She could concede the point either way.

Warmth gathered in their clasped hands as licks of Ollas's light burbled up to meet Eunny's. Their magic intertwined, settling around the cutting's leaves as she let their magic flow. He reached with his free hand to brush against a leaf. His fingers twitched reflexively, then dug into the soil.

With Ollas's magic spiraling around hers, Eunny followed suit, letting her palm settle atop the dirt as she urged a drop of her magic to bead at her fingertip. Ollas gave it a mental nudge, and the magic wicked through the substrate and spread through the branches in a glowing line to enter each unopened bud.

Eunny gasped. One by one, the dim glow in multiple buds went out. Snuffed like candles. Only, instead of a curl of smoke, they put out a wisp of golden light that hovered in the air as the little nubs dropped to the ground.

"Gently," Ollas murmured.

Together, they collected the tendrils of light with their joined hands, Eunny extending her index finger to catch each one. The wisps stuck to her skin, as fine as spider's silk. Ollas guided her hand to the base of the plant. With the help of Eunny's magic, he urged each strand to sink into the dirt. She poured more of her magic into the ground, reaching for whatever dregs she had left. Just as she had six years ago.

Except she wasn't alone this time. She didn't feel wobbles in her control. Exhaustion, yes, and a tingle of her old fear, too. That part hadn't completely left her.

Yet, when she called, her magic answered, just as it once had. Maybe not with the same force, but it traveled pathways the latent edges of her mind still remembered.

The remaining immature blossoms, only a trio or so left amongst the dark green leaves, began to swell. Tugging Ollas's magic along, Eunny cupped one of the buds between their palms. A velvety softness brushed against her skin. She lowered her hand so as not to inhibit the large, frilly, pink-and-red bloom. It kept spreading, rows of petals unfolding in a circular motion, wrinkling, and shriveling back as a new row opened in the center. The flower got to the size of Eunny's palm before the bloom withered a final time, sinking inward, its petals browning as they curled up.

Ollas carefully pulled the spent petals away to reveal a bulbous, green pod.

"I thought there were supposed to be—" A surprised squeak

that was not at all embarrassing came out of her when Ollas broke the pod open to reveal— "Seeds."

"It's not too late." Their gazes locked. "I don't think we've triggered the imprinting spell yet. We could give these to Ezzyn and Dae. They could take them to Rhell and you wouldn't have to bind yourself to them."

Eunny jerked her thumb toward the vine-covered door, where they could hear faint hacking and chopping. "Not leaving anything to chance. But if you want out, I won't stop you."

Ollas laughed, bending to give her a quick kiss. "Never."

"Good."

Eunny fed drops of their intertwined magic into the seeds, sighing with relief as she felt the minute pull of each of the over a dozen seeds drinking in some light. They vibrated briefly in her hand, attempting to pull more magic from their fingertips. Ollas's supply, always weak and flickery, petered out.

Panic fluttered in Eunny's belly. Her magic wavered as the reflex to shut it down, to rip out any semblance of the arcane from her mind and bury it beneath fear and denial and shame, roared through her head.

But those were the rash thoughts of Old Eunny. The woman who was content to run from her magic and convinced herself that that would be enough. That she could be happy with a mundane life.

Ollas gave her hand a reassuring squeeze.

Concentrating on the warmth of his palm against hers, the steadiness of his grip, Eunny exhaled with a measured breath.

Finally, she broke off her connection to the seeds.

They buzzed one last time, then went still. A tentative brush with just a whisper of her magic didn't cause them to stir. Eunny didn't get an impression of anything arcane in them at all.

The plant shuddered, its once-emerald leaves rapidly shriveling as they twisted and turned brown. The few remaining buds wrinkled and fell to the ground, their deep pink fading to a dusty taupe. Within seconds, the once-vibrant mini shrub was a withered husk of its former self.

Eunny glanced at Ollas, shoulders bobbing in a shrug. "That was close." She cupped the fresh seeds in her palm. Their brown shells had a deep, satiny shine. "I think it worked. They feel dormant or something."

"No!" Through a fist-sized hole in the vines, Bioon glared at them. "You wretched girl—"

In the distance, a horn call rang through the air. Ollas turned, peering through the misted glass of the antechamber's walls. "That's a Sentinel horn."

Bioon disappeared from the doorway.

Eunny leaned against the rack, sliding the new seeds into a discarded vial left near the door. She stared at the bedlam of the antechamber, the bits of vine and broken glass carpeting the floor. A laugh bubbled up in her throat. It came out maybe a tad hysterical, but she didn't care. She laughed anyway, knees going weak as adrenaline was replaced by fatigue and heady relief.

Ollas rubbed his sleeve against the smudged glass, not that it did much good. "I think I can see the others."

"That's wonderful. Get over here."

He glanced back at her. "Eh?"

He started to ask something, probably to see if she was okay, because he was kind and thoughtful like that—sweet words Eunny would never know, because they were lost to the depths of her mouth as she grabbed a fistful of his shirt and dragged him closer.

"Thank you," she murmured against his lips.

Ollas wrapped his arms around her. "Anything for my goddess."

"Anything?" Eunny drawled. "Goodness. What's a deity to do with so much power?"

His fingers kneaded her back, finding knots the excitement of the morning—gods all break, it was still only *morning*—had blissfully let her forget. "I can think of a few things," he said, lips traveling from her mouth to her neck.

"You and your greenhouse kink." Eunny's head tipped back. "I like—"

A knock on the glass made them look over.

"No fraternizing with the faculty," Dae called, her voice mock stern. "This is a school."

Laughing, Eunny made a rude gesture at her friend before pulling Ollas back for another kiss.

$$Chapter\ Twenty\text{-}Eight$$

THREE DAYS after the showdown in the greenhouse, Ollas found himself walking through the complex, once more bound for Trunk. The message board at the head of the complex was nearly bare, with only an informational poster about the various greenhouse hours stuck to a bottom corner. Soon enough, it would be covered with announcements for the fast-approaching Winterfest activities, and after that would come a fresh round of club openings and events and maybe a random call for housing in the spring term.

Cloak drawn about him to ward off the blessedly dry but cold air, Ollas slowed his step, taking in the neat, worn pathways tracing through the complex, the weathered paneling of the greenhouses, and the patina of age that turned the wooden frames a dark shade that was still warm and inviting. Quiet filled the air. Not silence, but gentle shifts and creaks brought on by rippling breeze. The Grove felt cozy and familiar and like home. Even though he'd only been back full time for one term, the place had always been with him.

Would it stay? He'd be leaving again, and not in the way of

upper-level studies where returning was relatively easy. He'd be gone, if not for good then at least for a while. Not so easy to stumble back to the Grove when homesickness struck if he was beyond the Valley's borders.

Eyes still roving over the board, he began to move on and nearly bumped into another person coming up the path. "Ah— Oh, sorry, sir—er, Saren."

Rai gave him a bemused look. "Ollas." He gestured with one hand. "Walk with me a moment."

"Of course," Ollas mumbled, falling into step beside him as Rai continued along the path.

Rai was wearing his teaching robes even though classes weren't in session, some dirt smudging the sleeves. In one hand he held a cutting from the Trunk's protector vine, secure in a glass vial filled with blue-tinted water. Strange for Ollas to be nervous now considering that they'd spent the last three months as colleagues. But then, being colleagues with a Master grovetender had always been a disconcerting notion for him.

"You've been busy," Rai said. "How are you holding up?"

"I, um, well, I think?"

"You think," Rai repeated.

"As well as can be expected. The school's been very... accommodating."

An understatement, and maybe even something of a dodge. Ollas wasn't in any trouble, formal or otherwise. When Ollas had offered to resign, seeing as he'd piqued the wrath of one of Graelynd's most powerful ruling bodies, the dean wouldn't hear of it. After giving his account of the events to Rai and the dean, he'd expected to be questioned by the school board, the Restorers, maybe even shipped down to Graelynd for gods-all-knew whatever reason to be grilled by Coalition folk or one of the Councils. Instead, the dean had told him to pack his bags and keep his head down for a while for everything to blow over. A sabbatical. It was laughable, considering he'd only been teaching for one term, but Ollas had taken the out, thanked the school, and negotiated seeing through his professional duties for his Initiate One class and the elective.

There was still much posturing going on with the Coalition, whispers of treasonous acts going on behind closed doors. He'd barely had a quiet moment with Eunny since they'd left the greenhouse, as she'd been involved not only in her own debriefings but also several long meetings that included her aunt. Whatever consequences were to be handed down to Bioon, he didn't know. But he'd faced down the notorious Coalition and come out unscathed.

Better than unscathed, because he had Eunny. She—*they*—had the seeds, and a fresh round of hope. His head was still spinning from the many turns of events.

"It's my understanding that you're being looked after by our good friends in Rhell," Rai said.

"I've had an offer to oversee a course at a school in Rhell," Ollas replied, staring straight ahead so he couldn't know his mentor's reaction. "Courtesy of the Sor'vahl family, no doubt, though the earth Magister in charge didn't mention them."

"Which subjects?"

"Arcane amendments and regenerative soil work."

The professor stopped at a crossroads in the path, opting for a bench instead of choosing a direction. "Sounds right in your wheelhouse."

Ollas sat next to him. "I've been very lucky. I feel kind of bad about it," he admitted, sheepish. "Undeserving."

Rai indicated the vine cutting in his hand. "A guardian wouldn't wake for nothing."

Ollas ran his fingertip along a single leaf. "Coincidence?"

"Greenhouses have been vandalized in the past. Disgruntled students. Tourists." Rai shrugged. "We once lost decades of work on a grain hybrid that had great promise for drought resistance, which we'd hoped to send south. An accidental fire destroyed everything in the antechamber. The guardians didn't intervene then."

"What makes them choose?"

"The quality of the need. The querent's intention. One can't say with certainty what the threshold is, but you met it." Rai smiled. "Miss Lee found a record in the archives that suggests the mother plant was a gift from Gyo the Earthen to Sylveren the Child when the Court began to leave the mortal realm. The motives of children aren't always—"

The wind kicked up, bringing with it a brief shower of icy rain.

"The gods weren't perfect," Rai continued in tones of mild annoyance. "They left for varied reasons, and we forge our own paths in their absence."

Another petulant gust of wind blasted them before settling down. Ollas hid a grin.

"So, you're bound for Rhell soon?" Rai asked.

"Yes, after finals." Provided Eunny agreed. Ollas realized that they hadn't actually discussed their plans, too busy with the aftermath of dealing with the Coalition. In the brief moments they'd been together, Eunny seemed enthusiastic about him sticking around, but, as he'd learned, presumptions instead of communication always led to problems. "I think."

"I could speak to the dean if you'd rather stay," Rai said. "I know you have family here, and you've only just returned. The Restorers approved a host of grants dedicated to the bioremediation research for Rhell's poison. Multiple Magister-levels are going to be putting together labs here at home."

"Thank you, but I can't stay," Ollas said, both touched and struck with a small pang of regret.

Rai sighed. "I was afraid you'd say that." He looked up at something, a serene smile on his face. "But I am not surprised. Be well, Ollas."

Ollas murmured his own farewell, turning to search for whatever the professor had seen. A smile spread across his own face, not serene but ebullient. Those little pangs of regret meant nothing when the sight of Eunny coming toward him brought such immediate joy.

"What was that about?" she asked, stopping in front of him.

"Goodbye, of a sort." Ollas stood up and wrapped his arms around her. "Come on. I— What's that?"

Eunny had fished from her cloak pocket the vial of their new delegation seeds. "Feels like we should do something. Memorialize them somehow."

The breeze picked up, swirling the hems of their cloaks about their legs.

"See?" she said. "The Valley agrees with me."

"Then we'll plant one. Maybe two, for luck." Ollas gestured at their surroundings. "Same place?"

She snorted. "I'd rather not. No light mage is meant to spend as much time in a greenhouse as I have this term."

Ollas chuckled. "You know, we're probably going to be doing greenhouse work in Rhell. This time of year, we won't be able to do in-ground planting until—"

Eunny clapped a hand over his mouth. "Don't ruin this for me."

He took her gently by the hand, pressing his lips to her curled fingers. "We've been talking about Rhell and plans and the work, but we didn't really— *I* never actually asked if this is what you want."

Her lopsided smile was followed by a soft laugh and a rueful shake of her head. "Gods, you're sweet. It's what I love about you." She cupped his face between her palms. "We're going. Together. Wouldn't have it any other way."

Same old Eunny, always moving forward. "I love you." Ollas tipped his chin forward to kiss her.

Eunny deepened the kiss, her fingers moving to his shoulders and grabbing handfuls of his cloak. She released him with an exaggerated sigh. "No, we have to focus. Memorialization in progress."

Ollas retrieved the vial from her, gently rubbing it between his fingers. He leaned toward her. "How do you feel about a little magic?"

The look she gave him was unimpressed, but she rolled her eyes and hooked her arm through his all the same.

They took the path back through the greenhouse complex, bypassing the buildings per Eunny's request. Ollas led her to the base of the Grove's mother tree, leaving the paved stone trails to settle in a spot between the massive roots. The ground was a mix of half-decayed leaf litter and patchy grass, and it was easy enough to work up shallow divots with a rake of his fingers. As Eunny had said, this wasn't planting so much as laying to rest. Tiny motes of light drifted down from the canopy of fiery leaves overhead, their magic keeping the mighty tree always full and lush no matter the season. Many of the gleaming dots dissipated before they reached the floor, but every once in a while, one made it, fading out in a small ripple of white-gold light.

"This is..." Eunny held her hand out to catch a drop of the Grove's light, smiling as it absorbed into her skin. "Perfect."

"Ready?" he asked.

She called a touch of light to her fingers, holding her hand in front of her face. "I'm still not sure how I feel about it. It's going to be a while before I'm comfortable using it again."

"I can do it," he offered. "I think I have enough."

She shook her head. "Together. I can't let discomfort keep being an excuse."

Eunny knelt, tapping a pair of seeds into her cupped palm. Ollas joined her, and together, they called a touch of light to their fingers. He slid his palm around to cradle her hand, letting her magic meld with his until it blurred together. Eunny directed the lines of their combined light to pool in her hand and settle on the seeds. Ollas drew on his wavering magic, helped along by Eunny's steadier supply, causing the seeds to flare with soft, golden outlines.

Gently, Eunny tilted her palm until the seeds could fall into the shallow hole Ollas had made. They landed with minute tremors, disappearing as Ollas smoothed soil back over the top. Watering them in would've been ideal, but the ground was wet enough, and it would only be a matter of hours before the next rain shower came through.

As they dusted off their hands, a faint puff of white sparks drifted up from the ground. A soft pulse beat at Ollas's temple, just once, but enough that memory stirred. The old calling that had been with him since the summer echoed in his head before fading away.

A glance at Eunny confirmed that she'd felt the same thing. She scrunched her nose at him in mock disgruntlement. "Guess it thought we needed the reminder that we're in this for the long haul."

A gust of wind scattered the sparks throughout the air, carrying them up toward the treetops. Eunny and Ollas watched until the sparks were lost to sight.

"Think it was wrong to waste two here when we're about to leave?" she asked.

Ollas shook his head. "Now a little of them is here, and the main seeds are going to Rhell. Doesn't get more fitting than that." He helped her to her feet, one hand smoothing her hair from her face. "Feel ready for a new journey?"

Eunny laughed. She took him by the hand and tugged him back toward the road. "Almost. There's one last goodbye." A wicked gleam twinkled in her eyes. "And I want to hear the final judgment for my mother."

Chapter Twenty-Nine

THE FEELING of cold metal against her bare skin made a shiver run down Eunny's spine. She ignored it. Fingers wrapped around the blades to keep them firmly closed, she offered the small shears to Gransen, handle first.

"Honor's all yours," she said, wiggling the handle when Gransen could only stare at her. "Granse. *Manage.*"

He startled, a grin breaking across his face. "Can't believe you're doing this."

"Me either, believe me," she grumbled. A wry smile threatened to ruin her cool façade. "Go on. You deserve it."

Taking the shears, Gransen set the open edge against the plain woven ribbon. It was still a little stained at the edges, but several washes—not to mention a dye bath to turn it from grubby beige to a deep red—had gotten rid of the musty smell. And what better than a reclaimed and repaired ribbon to commemorate the grand reopening of Song's Scrap?

With a hearty snip, the shears cut through the ribbon, and the two halves fluttered to the ground. A cheer went up from the crowd gathered in the street. Gransen flung open the new double doors, giving a dramatic bow as he cried, "Song's Scrap is officially open for business!"

Eunny stepped back, parking herself off to the side of the entryway. She nodded and murmured thanks to the townsfolk; those she was friendly with stopped by for a quick word. She'd been surprised to find a few dozen folks attending the repair café's opening but had figured most were just there out of communal goodwill or idle curiosity. Winter in Sylvan was relatively slow outside of Winterfest activities, and they still had a few blessed weeks of quiet before the holiday machine started up. Now that the ribbon was cut, Eunny assumed people would opt for food and drink at the Mighty Leaf.

Many did, but to her surprise, a good many did *not*, instead shuffling through the repair café's doors. Some clutched their own items, intent on making use of the café's services. Terryl Nevin led a small group of her fellow library staff, their hands full with assorted sewing and other needlework projects.

Terryl swept Eunny up in a hug, murmuring in her ear, "Olly's in line at the teashop," before following her colleagues to the main table by the window.

Several people, mostly visitors, merely went in to see what the café had to offer, politely nodding in greeting as they went past. Eunny looked to the side, where the salvaged metal sign hung once more from the roof. A new, smaller one had been added underneath, announcing *Song's Scrap, Owner—Eunny Song, Managed by Gransen Mast.*

"It looks good. Legitimate," Dae said, coming up beside Eunny.

Calya and Zhenya joined them. "Who knew this heap could clean up so nice," Calya added.

Eunny scoffed, bumping the younger woman with her shoulder.

"Is that any way to treat an ally?" Calya groused when, by

trying to escape, she stepped in a puddle. Perhaps the brief gust of wind that kicked up on what was otherwise a calm day had helped. "This place hates me. I'm leaving soon enough, okay?" she said in exasperation to the sky.

"Are you okay, though?" Eunny asked, voice lowering.

"No, now my feet are wet for my nausea-inducing ride home."

Dae sighed. "Caly."

Calya gave an indifferent shrug. "Nothing I can't handle."

"Don't get into shit with the Coalition on my account," Eunny said.

"Bit late for that, isn't it?"

"Then fix it. Apologize. I can try and—"

Calya dismissed Eunny's words with a wave of her hand. "No. They have no legal quarrel with me." Her lips spread with a predator's smile. "Besides, it's good for the Coalition to know not every business in Graelynd will be cowed by them."

Dae rubbed her hand over her face. "My baby sister. Taking on the Scourge of Graelynd."

Eunny and Zhenya exchanged glances, but the younger woman only shrugged. When it came to managing Helm Naval, Calya had always been headstrong. Eunny hadn't expected her to outright lie to the Coalition members en route to the Valley, but the younger Helm daughter had done...almost that. Embroiled Bioon's colleagues in HNE affairs regarding the investigation into the Brint Avenor debacle from earlier in the year. The finer details of her dealings with the Coalition were known only to Calya herself. Eunny suspected the younger woman liked it that way, and would endeavor to keep the exact truth a mystery.

Eunny had wondered why her mother had showed up at the greenhouse with only two guards. Apparently, Calya's machinations had led to the detainment of the Coalition cohort in

Renstown. She had also forced the hand of the Sentinels investigating said cohort, but it had resulted in the recovery of the stolen delegation plants. The specimens had withered to desiccated husks as the bloom cycle ended unfulfilled, but the evidence was damning all the same. And Valley folk, even those in the larger town across the lake, didn't take kindly to Graelynders making demands and acting like they were above the laws of the Valley.

A group of Sentinels made their way into the Mighty Leaf. One of them noticed Eunny and her friends standing in front of the café and stopped. His hood was pulled back, revealing dark brown hair that fell past his shoulders. A frown marred his weather-tanned face, his gaze focused on Calya.

As if she felt his stare, Calya lifted her head, eyes seeking its origin. She returned the man's animosity with a pointed look of her own. The Sentinel turned away and vanished into the tearoom.

"What was that about?" Eunny asked as they all turned to Calya with expectant looks.

"Nothing. He was the Sentinels' liaison with the Coalition." She shrugged. "Suffice it to say, he should stick to being a woodsman. One needs a fast head for their business."

Before anyone could respond, the door to the Mighty Leaf opened again, and Bioon walked out, followed by her Coalition colleagues and a different escort of Sentinels. She stopped, then motioned toward Eunny. "I'd like a moment with my daughter, if you please."

When one of the Graelynders tried to protest, Bioon silenced him with a cold look.

"It's okay," Eunny said to her friends. "Go inside. This won't take long."

She followed her mother away from the buildings to a short outcropping that overlooked the road leading down to

Sylvan's small port. As they passed the Mighty Leaf, Eunny glanced inside to see Yerina standing at the counter, watching. It was hard to tell through the window, but Eunny thought her aunt looked... resolved. Wistful, but free of the kind of pained sadness that usually followed family interactions.

Standing close enough for conversation while still maintaining the distance of strangers, mother and daughter faced the water, unspeaking. Down in the harbor, a small windrunner, the type that held scarcely more than fifty passengers plus crew, was being readied to sail. Bioon would be on it soon, leaving Sylvan's shores in disgrace. The Coalition faced heavy sanctions and formal investigations for its transgressions, from both the Order of Sylveren and Graelynd's Upper Council, and Bioon had been stripped of her position in the organization. Seeing as neither Bioon nor any Coalition representatives were allowed in the Valley without express permission, Eunny realized it might be the last time she saw her mother in this place again. Probably the last time they would speak in a good long while, for Bioon was being reassigned to a backwater posting in southern Graelynd.

In the three days since the showdown at the greenhouse, Eunny had learned that Yerina had kept her promise to stall Bioon. Bioon had already been in Sylvan when she'd learned of her team's delay, and was prepared to charge up to the school when her sister insisted they talk. Sweet Yerina, the older sister who'd always been the pushover. Always so kind in the face of Bioon's chill. A lifetime of being sisters, and Yerina only gave and asked nothing in return. She'd finally come to collect, buying Eunny several precious minutes before her mother had seen the tactic for what it was and left. To have been fooled by *Yerina* of all people—for Bioon, there was no coming back from that.

"You handled yourself well up here, Eunji," her mother finally said. "You won your silly little seeds."

Those *silly little seeds* had dragged Bioon's ass up to the Valley. The Coalition had been willing to commit treason over them. A betrayal with the best of intentions, the Coalition had pled, a tepid agreement with the Eyllic Empire to try and adapt their poison so it could penetrate the Valley's arcane protections. In exchange, Eylle would share the secret of how they'd created their own magical wellspring, being the only nation to ever have managed such a feat. With Graelynd reliant on the abundant overflow from the Valley's wellspring, Eunny could begrudgingly admit to understanding the Coalition's interest. The seeds had been a guarantee of safety for the Coalition, providing plants that could be used to keep researchers from falling ill while they worked. The Coalition claimed their intent was to study the poison and provide an antidote for all. At a reasonable price, of course.

Only the Eyllics had changed the deal, withholding their supposed method of creating a wellspring until after the Coalition delivered. The empire had refused to allow any of the delegation to leave until agreements were made, sealed in blood. It was pure luck that Ollas's group of Sentinels had found them when they did, and after years at war, with Graelynders being held under threat of violence, it was easy to send the camp into chaos. The Coalition had destroyed as much evidence as they could linking them to such treachery. Might've gotten away with it, too, if not for a curious gardener planting some seemingly nondescript little brown seeds in an unused patch of ground on Sylveren's campus.

"Was it worth it, Mother? Betraying your allies, selling your soul."

"Don't get cute with me," Bioon said mildly. "And, yes. My only regret is that I failed."

"You can't be serious! Working with *Eylle*?"

"Nothing has stopped them so far, Eunji. Nothing. It's only a matter of time before they find a way to destroy the Valley, and then where will Graelynd be?" Bioon said, a fervent note in her tone that Eunny had never heard before. "Hate my methods, but you are too smart to not see the logic behind our work."

"The Coalition dumped you. No need to keep singing their praises."

"We have always acted in the best interests of Graelynd. The Coalition will always endeavor to protect her, to make the hard call so others can—"

"The Eyllic warlord won't rest until all the wellsprings are dust. You really think he'd leave Graelynd alone?" Eunny demanded. "Spare me your supposed patriotism. The Coalition wanted to make money. That's all it ever cares about."

Bioon gave a delicate shrug. "Believe what you like. Cling to your naïve hope. When the truth of Eylle's might is on your precious Valley's doorstep, perhaps you'll believe your mother then."

"They're hiding behind their walls across the sea. Think about that while you're checking timesheets or whatever scut work you've got to look forward to down in South District."

Behind them, Ollas called Eunny's name. She turned, raising her hand to wave.

"We've already got a way to stop the poison from spreading." Eunny grinned with teeth. "Now we can keep it from sickening people. I'd say things are looking up."

"For the sake of the Empyrean Territories, I hope that's true," Bioon murmured. "Do not be blinded by your pride, Eunji. The Coalition has resources—"

Eunny faced her mother. "You don't write. You *can't* visit. Let's keep it that way. For good."

Bioon said nothing, but there was a tightness to her smirk.

Eunny turned away, only to look back once more. "And Bioon? If you ever try to manipulate me again, or threaten Auntie Yerina, I will become your daughter. I'll fight as fucking dirty as you do." She held up her hand and summoned a palmful of light. "Remember that I never really lost my magic. That I have it and you don't. I'm the Healer Who Hurts, and I won't think twice about hurting you, *Mother*."

"Are you done?" Bioon said, her bored tone too forced to be authentic. "We sail within the hour."

Eunny turned, catching the eye of the lead guard responsible for escorting the Coalition to the docks and seeing them into Graelynd's custody. She nodded once, walking away from her mother without looking back.

"Are you okay?" Ollas asked as she stepped into his waiting arms.

"Never better," she said. "Just dumping some old baggage."

Ollas draped his arm around her, shivering dramatically as he squeezed her close. "Can we go inside? It's freezing out here, and Yerina made those melty cheese bun things."

Eunny laughed, letting him steer her back toward the café. "We leave for Rhell in a few days, to spend most of the winter in the north. This is nothing."

"It's a good thing I'll have you to keep me warm."

"What happened to worshipping at the Altar of Song?" Eunny said with mock indignation. "Goddesses don't do all the work."

"I will happily do the work." Ollas kissed the side of her head, lips lingering by her ear. "We'll both be nice and warm, I promise."

With a big, silly grin on her face, Eunny took him by the hand and pulled him back into her shop.

<h1 style="text-align:center">Epilogue</h1>

Despite a few trying moments of late, Ollas still considered himself something of an optimist. Usually, being a believer didn't steer him astray. Not too badly, at least.

"Are you sure?" Eunny held the last word, laughter and a hint of a challenge in her tone. "I can amuse myself until you get back."

Ollas glanced at the wall clock. He had to squint to read the fancy indicators so many Rhellian timekeepers favored. Both the design of the face and the hands leaned more toward art than practicality. "I've got time."

Always. He'd always have time for his personal goddess. Would make it, if necessary. When she was tense or frustrated about her renewed relationship with magic, he was there. A shoulder to lean on, or a hand to hold in quiet support. And the days when she needed to vent about the latest change Gransen had made in the running of the repair café? Ollas lent his ear.

And for mornings such as this, when Eunny felt a particular sort of hunger an hour—less than, actually, if he'd read the clock correctly—before his first day of teaching at Triune,

Rhell's premier college? He could offer her a few options of amenable body parts for perusal. The advantages of faculty housing and a small campus.

"The building's not too far from here." Ollas slipped his tunic over his head. "I'll run." The rest of his clothes joined the tunic on the floor.

Eunny scoffed with mild disbelief. It didn't stop her from rummaging in the nightstand for a contraceptive potion. "Showing up late, sweaty, and out of breath on your first day. Your students will be aghast."

"I won't be la-*late*." His breath caught as she took him firmly in hand and pulled him closer to the bed.

With very little prompting, Ollas tumbled to the mattress. No sooner had he rolled onto his back than Eunny straddled him. She still wore her night slip. Only her night slip, he couldn't help but notice, as she slowly ground against him. How she *slid*. Clearly, someone had already been amusing herself this morning while Ollas went about his final prep work. Not that he was complaining. Besides, he rather liked the garment. It draped over her frame, the material so soft, so sheer, that it left nothing to imagination.

"Remind me again how you got out of having anything to do with a class focusing on growing *our* seeds?" Ollas asked, his hands settling on her hips.

"I don't teach." Eunny reached for the bottle of lubricant and put a few drops on her fingers. "And it's not *nothing*. I'll be there once you're doing the hands-on stuff."

"Sure, but they're—"

She wrapped her fingers around his cock and gave it a rough pump.

Ollas moaned. "That was mean."

"I didn't sign myself up for school. Again." Eunny ran her

thumb over his cockhead, smearing the bead of pre-come gathered at the tip. "Any more questions, Professor?"

He shook his head.

"Good boy." She leaned down to press her lips against his in a deceptively gentle kiss. "I'll be quick. Since you're in a rush."

"You don't need to—"

The rest of his words, his thoughts, were lost as Eunny rose up on her knees and sank onto him. His suspicions were proven correct; she had prepared herself for him. As much as she was able, anyway, with her beautiful, graceful, *thin* mender's fingers. Enough that she could take half of his cock on her first try before she stilled and gave him a squeeze with her inner walls.

Ollas groaned. His cock throbbed with the need to go farther, deeper. None of this halfway shit. Eunny's pussy was sinful, the perfect blend of tight yet yielding. It beckoned, urged him to press in. Ollas didn't know how, but he'd swear on the Earthen's shrine that she did it on purpose, as if she knew how to make herself have *just* enough give. The kind that tempted an awkward little bean with gallant intentions to forget himself and plow her into the bed.

He gripped her waist, tugging with small, innocuous motions as his hips began to rise.

Eunny swatted at his hands. "Behave." She rose up until only his tip remained, desperate, inside of her. "Or I'll send you off to class while I enjoy the bag of fun times Gransen gave us."

The most piteous sound came out of Ollas's mouth, but he let his hands drop, and his ass went flat on the bed.

With a self-satisfied hum, Eunny began to move. She sank onto him again, sitting back on her heels as much as she could. She rose up and did it again, and again, a little faster each time. A little farther. She started to pause, sometimes at his tip, other times when she had most of his length snugly held, and give him a squeeze.

Constrained by her warning, and threat, Ollas only allowed himself minimal—so small he could blame it on the natural motion of the bed—thrusts to meet her more purposeful ones. But when she began to tighten around him, her eyes closing, head tipping back as she finally could lower herself flush against his groin, his control disintegrated. He was hard enough to burst with just a tiny bit of prompting, his body trembling with the pressure of holding himself back. A slight change of angle, tap her in the right place, and he could—

"Wait for me," Eunny said between gasps.

Ollas groaned. He needed to touch her. Something, anything to sate the urge for roughness without defying her command. His fingers crept along her thighs, not pulling down but grasping merely to feel her flesh in his hands. Her eyes pinched shut again, her breaths soft moans. Her nipples had formed points, poking at the thin slip. Gods, but did he love the way her tits bounced when she rode him. Loved her enthusiasm. Everything about her, really, even the sweet torture she put him through.

Finally, she collapsed forward, her hands going to his shoulders as she used him for leverage. He slid his palms over the curve of her ass, and he couldn't help himself but to let his fingers grab hold. When she shifted, making her shapely muscle flex in his hands, Ollas was done for.

"Now, love? Please?" he begged.

Eunny nodded.

His grip on her ass tightened. His pelvis canted up to meet her as she bore down. A few short, deep bucks into her, tilting her just enough for a light bit of friction against her clit, and she was gone. Her pussy fluttered around him, enveloping his cock with a series of contractions felt all throughout his body. It was bliss, easily enough to get Ollas to let himself go. His balls drew tight as his thrusts stuttered. His cock pulsed alongside her clenching waves, his climax adding his own brand of heat.

She flopped on top of him, smiling against his chest when he grunted in weak protest. She reached up, batting around until she found his cheek and gave it a pat. "You better get running."

Ollas nuzzled the side of her neck, drunk on her musk. "Don't bathe."

"Ever?" She snorted, rolling off him and onto her back.

"Until after class." He scooted down so he could position himself between her thighs. The sight of his spend, creamy white against her dark, slickened folds, made something deep and primal rumble in his chest. "No, you're right. Never is best."

His seed threatened to leak out. Ollas pressed it back in, entranced by the sight of his fingers burying his come inside of her.

"Nev!" Eunny yelped as his thumb circled her clit. "You're going to be late."

Ollas glanced at the clock. "I'll sprint."

Fresh off her first orgasm, she didn't need any more warming up. He shoved three fingers in her as he lowered his mouth to her clit.

"*Nev!*" Eunny's back arched as her hips tried to dance away, but Ollas wrapped his free arm around her leg to keep her in place. His fingers worked her over, not ruthless but, as he liked to think of it, efficient. In their relatively short time together, he had dedicated himself to learning the precise pleasures of his goddess. After all, he believed in the value of a good education.

Eunny squirmed as his tongue lapped at her most sensitive part. He tasted some of the odd slipperiness of the lubricant, a bit of his tang and salt, but mostly her sweetness. It did some-thing to his brain, made him almost tingly numb with pleasure, a sensation only eclipsed by the feeling of her writhing as she came again on his fingers.

Ollas pressed a soft kiss to her clit, then nipped at her thigh, grinning when she whined. He slid away. "Remember about the bath."

He performed the fastest, probably-not-very-effective washup while also dashing around their small apartment, yanking on clothes. Fuck, he *was* going to be late. Worth it, but not a great look for his first day. Thank the gods they'd be outside today, doing a ground assessment.

"Nev." Eunny sat cross-legged on the bed. She beckoned him closer with the crook of a finger. "Your tunic is on backwards."

"Shit." He went over to her, dragging his arms through the armholes so she could reorient the garment.

Instead of fixing his clothes, Eunny rose up on her knees, one arm snaking around his neck to pull his head closer. She kissed him, slowly, letting her fingers trail down his front.

"Eun—" Ollas tried to speak, but her tongue slid into his mouth. Arms pinned by his clothing, he was helpless to stop her roving hand. He supposed he could've stepped away, but no part of his traitorous body entertained the thought seriously. In truth, he was all too willing to return her kisses. Lean into her touch. One particular part of him was ready to skive off silly things like professional responsibility and prior commitments in favor of falling back into bed.

She gripped his cock through the front of his trousers, coaxed it back to hard in just a few firm strokes. Sucked his lower lip into her mouth, humming so sweetly to him. The sound and pressure made Ollas tremble, a shiver running down his spine. Down his cock. It bobbed against her hand as an ache settled in his balls. Eunny smiled against his lips.

Then she abruptly drew back. "If I have to wait in discomfort"—she spun his tunic around to the correct position and tapped his chest—"so do you."

"What?" Ollas said, dazed.

She peered down at him, at the tent his cock was trying to pitch in his trousers. She grinned, nudging him toward the door. "Get going."

Ollas moaned. Forget sprinting; he'd need to sprout wings to get there in time.

Still grumbling, he kissed her hard and quick, maybe even a tad petulant. With a pointed look, he flipped his cock up behind his waistband and stumbled out the door.

THE END

Thank you for reading *Growing Memories*. I hope you enjoyed Eunny and Ollas's happy ending. Please consider telling a friend or leaving a review on your platform of choice— It truly is one of the best ways you can support a book!

Did Ollas's greenhouse kink rub off on you? Join my monthly newsletter and receive access to the nsfw art piece of the scene from Chapter 19.

Sign up for my newsletter here!

NEXT IN THE VALLEY OF SYLVEREN

The fight against the Eyllic poison concludes with Calya and Nocren in *Mistral Hearts (Valley of Sylveren #3)*.

THE VALLEY OF SYLVEREN TRILOGY

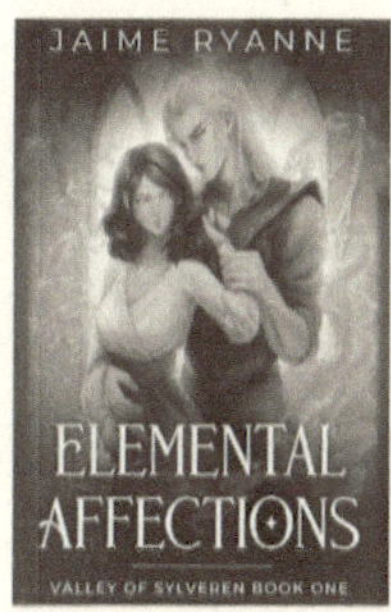
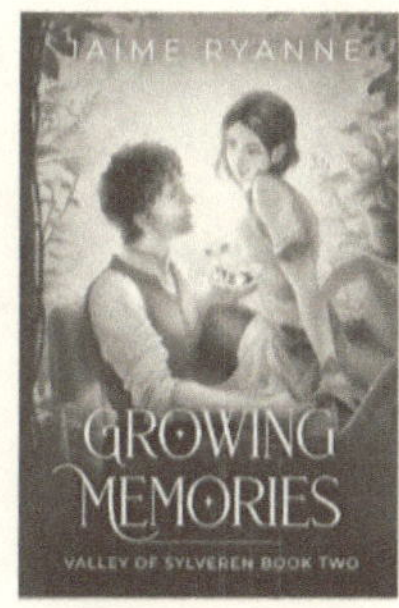
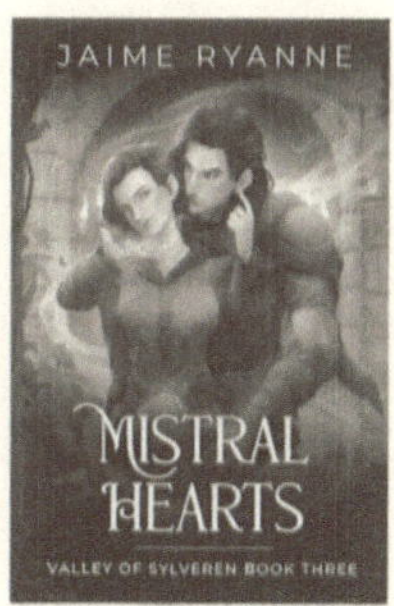

The story concludes with:

MISTRAL HEARTS

A diviner who's sworn off romance. An heiress who's all business. Fate brings them together, but the fear of love could drive them apart.

Acknowledgments

Well, we made it. The middle child of the Valley of Sylveren trilogy is done, and hopefully you, dear reader, enjoyed your time with Eunny, Ollas, and the rest of the gang. I know I did... sort of. This book was a rollercoaster to write, and we might not have made it to the end without the patience and support of my husband, Steven. Thank you, hon, for keeping the cats entertained while I tried to write, for putting up with my angst over this book—even before the Wrist Incident that dialed the stress up to 11, and enduring far too many "Ok, I've revised the outline and now I *really* think it's going to work. I'm happy with it." (It did not, dear reader, and I was not. Every time.)

Thanks as always to Cara, for being my #1 hype guy and supplying me with an endless amount of silly reels to keep me out of the depths of despair. Thank you for also being super supportive, and forever willing to take up the mantle when Steven said, "I don't know, ask Cara."

Thank you to my critique partners: Cara M., Marit H., Kelley F., Rhoda B., and Steven M., for your wonderful, thoughtful feedback. You are all amazing, and I appreciate you to bits. I am so fortunate that our paths managed to cross, and my words are the better for it. An extra shoutout to Marit, for many things, but especially for saving my ass when it came to the herbalism in this book. Any inaccuracies or nonsensical parts are completely my own. (But also, dear reader, this book is fiction, not medical advice.)

Many hands are involved in making a book go from ideas in

my head to something you can hold in your hands. Thank you to Isla Elrick and Adie Hart for their insight and eagle eyes in the editing and proofreading, and being so incredibly accommodating when the Wrist Incident of late April necessitated a lot of reshuffling. Thank you to Sarah C., for being a great PA with impeccable organizational skills and the added bonus of lots of tips for dealing with a wrecked wrist. You're truly full service! Thanks to my wonderful street team, for the hype and the love; you all continue to amaze and thrill me with your creativity. And thank you to Jin (Zureiil), for the absolutely amazing cover. It's a dream come true to have your art as the face of my books.

To my friends and family, thank you for your love and excitement about my books, for celebrating their existence, and for not allowing my introverted self to stay (as) quiet about them. I see what you're doing, and it is greatly appreciated.

And finally, thank you to my readers. I'll always be a writer, but I couldn't publish like this without you.

Jaime Ryanne, June 2025

The Valley of Sylveren

Elemental Affections

Growing Memories

Mistral Hearts

The World of Sylveren

A New Leaf

www.jaimeryanne.com/books

About the Author

JAIME RYANNE writes fantasy romance featuring competent heroines of color, secondary world settings with modern touches, and plenty of spice. There's usually angst involved, but it always comes with a happy ending.

She is a Korean American adoptee living in the Pacific Northwest with her husband and two cats. When she isn't writing, if she's sitting then she's probably knitting (or spinning yarn. Actual yarn, not tales). She loves fountain pens, collecting notebooks, and wishes her enthusiasm for gardening was reflected in the actual results.

www.jaimeryanne.com
Instagram: @jaimeryanne_writes